What others are saying about this book:

"This book found me at home nursing my first child through an illness. What a revelation! How wonderful it was to read such a message of nurturance as [...] new role as caregiver. It changed th[...]

"This book invites us to listen intimately and gently to the body and healing process, teaching beyond dogma to a celebration of a prayerful relationship with life."

— Alison Hine, MSW, *therapist, spiritual director*

"In an age when more and more individuals are wanting to take responsibility for their own health and well-being, this practical handbook offers an excellent starting place. Combining the best of both alternative and allopathic approaches, it offers personal examples plus a clear guide to seeking professional care."

— Paul Dugliss, M.D., Director, Oakwood Complementary and Alternative Medicine Center

"... Sandra and Leo are wholly committed to nurturing the bodies and souls of each other and their four children, and there is much wisdom in the pages of this book. I know it will guide my family and many others on a path toward wholeness."

— *homeschooling mother, active member of La Leche League*

"...While suffering from the side effects of cancer therapy, I accumulated many herbs and remedies never fully understanding how to use them. *Healing at Home* brings it all together in a clear, gentle, and caring guide. Valuable gifts can come about through illness, if we are wise enough to accept them."

— *artist, cancer survivor*

Healing at Home

A Guide to Using Alternative
Remedies and Conventional Medicine
That Will Change Your Approach to
Illness

Sandra Greenstone

with Clinton L. Greenstone, M.D.

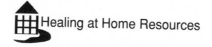Healing at Home Resources

Published by: 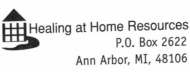 Healing at Home Resources
P.O. Box 2622
Ann Arbor, MI, 48106
e-mail: lindo@compuserve.com

Copyright © 1999, Sandra Greenstone

All rights reserved. No part of this publication may be reproduced, stored in a retrieval system or transmitted in any form or by any means, without prior written permission from the author. Requests to the publisher may be submitted to the address listed above.

Every effort has been made to trace the ownership of all copyrighted material. If any omission has been made, please contact the publisher, so that proper acknowledgment may be given in future editions.

Grateful acknowledgment is made for permission to reprint portions of the following copyrighted material. *Caring for the Sick at Home* by T. Bentheim, and *A Guide to Child Health* by Michaela Gloekler and Wolfgang Goebel copyright by Anthroposophic Press.

Disclaimer

This book is intended to educate people about a variety of approaches to healthcare needs. The information contained in this book is not intended to serve as a replacement for the personal care and treatment of a qualified physician, but rather should be used in conjunction with a physician's care. Any use of the information in this book is at the reader's discretion. The author and the publisher specifically disclaim any and all liability arising directly from the use or application of any information contained in this book. If you do not wish to be bound by the above, you may return this book for a full refund.

Edited by: Rahima Baldwin Dancy, Margo Von Minden

Layout Design and Typesetting: Shannon Feldt (Berger)

Illustrations: Sandra Greenstone

Cover Design: Tim Feldges

Library of Congress Catalog Card Number: 99-94425

ISBN: 0-9671863-0-7

ABOUT THE AUTHORS

Sandra Greenstone comes from a small town in northern Canada. She has spent much of her life healing from a potentially life-threatening illness. For over twenty years she has been studying and living holistic healing and is a certified practitioner of Process Acupressure.

She also has an extensive academic and professional background in communications and media, specializing as a producer of health-related documentary film.

Clinton L. Greenstone, M.D. received his medical degree from Yale University and completed his training in Internal Medicine at UC San Francisco. He is currently a Clinical Assistant Professor of Medicine at the University of Michigan and the Medical Director of Oakwood Healthcare System's Complementary and Alternative Medicine Center in Westland, Michigan. He has spent most of his career studying, practicing, and teaching human-centered medicine.

Together they live in a co-housing community where they are parenting, homeschooling, and "healing at home" with their four very young children.

ACKNOWLEDGMENTS

Many wise and loving souls have participated in the birth of this book including colleagues, clients, community members, friends, and family. I thank you all. It was your generous feedback and insights that ultimately kept me going and brought this book to life. (Marcia, Ellen and Scott, Diana, Iris and Doug, Rowena, J.D. and Carol, Doug and Claudia, Nina, Mary Lynn, Mary, Tim and Jo-Ann and the whole Feldt clan. Also, M. Dobson, P. Incao, MD, R. Baldwin Dancy, C. & F. Murphy, M. Von Minden, P. Dugliss, MD, G. Karnow, MD, and J. Worzniak, MD.)

I would especially like to thank:

My husband, Leo, for his enduring love and consistent willingness to wrangle with our ideas and hearts to find the unified path that resulted in this book.

Shannon Feldt, whose creativity and ability to relentlessly "keep trying" sustained me as we sailed through the uncharted waters of this process, revision after endless revision.

Andrea Rentea, whose strong and caring presence planted the seed 10 years ago.

Aminah Raheem, for the love and healing teachings she brings to the world.

My four ever-loving children, Nya, Jackson, Miles and Stanton. You inspire me to heal and grow everyday. Without you, this book would not exist. Because of you, it almost didn't.

TABLE OF CONTENTS

1

YOUR GUIDE TO RECLAIMING THE HEALING PROCESS

Welcome to the healing revolution! Millions of people are searching for new and more inclusive ways to understand and work with health and illness. With the comforting advice of a doctor, this book offers you just that. The basic organization of this book and companion healing kit will teach you how to navigate your way through most common illnesses and injuries while strengthening your healing potential. You can also become more self-reliant by learning how and when to use home therapies, natural medicines, and pharmaceutical drugs. And when unexpected injuries and illnesses develop, you can have all the necessary healing substances at your fingertips in a healing kit.

This project came from our family's attempt to simplify and make sense of an overwhelming amount of information, products, and healthcare options. Our healing kit and book sit together in a cupboard above the fridge in one handy little box. From slivers and cuts to fevers and flus, this approach has taken much of the chaos, fear, and frustration out of healing at home.

THE GUIDE

This is a practical and powerful guide to supporting the healing process. It is a guide to the parameters of safe home care and to choosing and combining the most appropriate paths of healing. It also offers ways to promote a healing life-style. In case of an illness or injury, it suggests how to support the body's own innate healing forces through rest, rhythm, caring for the senses, fluids, warmth, nutrition, and massage. Finally, there are three quick reference sections on common illnesses, basic first aid, and home therapies and information on how and why to use them.

The guide is a blend of information derived from homeopathic, anthroposophic, herbal, eastern, and mainstream western medicine. It can help you build bridges between these modalities, depending on the situation and the condition.

This bridging is greatly inspired by Dr. Rudolf Steiner's indications through anthroposophical medicine, which views the human being and illness as an interconnected whole, combining body, mind, emotions, and spirit. It is an approach that views illness as the human experience of a disease and healing as stemming from the word holy, or to become whole. As you learn to see the connection between your body, thoughts, relationships, and behaviors, you unleash the potential for a greater sense of well-being, sense of purpose, and joy in your life.

This guide helps answer questions like:

Does this person need immediate medical attention?

How can I support the person's own healing forces?

What home therapies can be used to assist the healing?

When and how do I need to use them?

How can I be sure these natural medicines are working?

Do I have them on hand or in a kit?

What do I watch for to know that the healing process is in place?

When are commonly prescribed drugs necessary, and what is their role?

What warning symptoms do I watch for to indicate the need for medical care?

How do I care for myself as the caregiver?

These symptoms keep happening again and again. What is the pattern and what is the meaning of this illness?

Is this symptom a hassle or a blessing? Is there a connection between illness, healing, and human development?

THE HEALING KIT

You can purchase a ready-made kit or create your own.

The ready-made kit includes the essential herbs, natural medicines, essential oils, and ointments mentioned in this book. The kit also provides extra spaces for you to add pharmaceuticals, thermometer, bandages, and other healing supplies. This gives you quick access to the things you wish you had "on hand", while leaving room for tailoring the kit to your unique needs. To order, see the "Healing Kit" information page at the back of the book.

If you already have some of these home remedies or prefer using others, that's great. Many of the basic principles will still apply to what you already have and may inspire you to create your own healing kit.

THE POINT

This is more than a simple reference guide to home therapies for common illnesses. The core message is that healing happens mostly through the way we live and the way we respond to illness. Supporting the healing process, as outlined in Section Five, is the single most important way to promote healing in the case of any illness or injury. Using commonly prescribed drugs and home therapies can merely assist in this process.

Also, while you read this guide, let it be an exercise in listening to yourself. Let it inspire you to pay attention to your symptoms, observe your patterns, and go within more deeply than you have. This is where the gold is. This is where the journey to healing begins.

Finally, there is also a deeper purpose or motivation in healing. The healthier and more joyful we become, the more we are able to serve our communities and support one another in this grand process of human evolution.

2

PERSONAL PATH TO HEALING

THE WAKE UP CALL

At age 10 I noticed that I had difficulty peeling potatoes and complained of aching knees. I was diagnosed with juvenile rheumatoid arthritis, an illness that runs in my family. I was immediately hospitalized to control the swelling. I began a pharmaceutical regimen of 12 aspirin a day, myochrisine or liquid gold injections, and extensive physical therapy.

I was an extremely active young child and my symptoms were rather mild. So this felt like a little holiday from school, and I enjoyed the extra attention. However, during physical therapy I befriended several girls my age who had the same disease. They were not ice skating or playing the piano or soccer like I was. I didn't see them laugh or smile much either. Their joints were very deformed; they walked with crutches or were confined to wheelchairs; they looked much older than they were; and they taught me how to inject the stinging gold liquid into my thighs every day. This was the wake up call.

At age 18 I started working at a health food store and reading about alternative ways of working with physical healing. My focus at that point was on nutrition and exercise. My symptoms stabilized and I went into remission for several years.

THE ALARM

I was 22, in the final year of my undergraduate degree. I was not very happy. I had slowly stopped taking care of myself. The place where I was working felt awful. The building felt awful. The skirt and panty hose I was wearing felt awful. My relationships felt empty. I felt like I was trying to prove myself to my family and the world. I questioned the meaning of my entire university experience. I felt like I was just going through the motions. I was living in my head.

One morning I woke up with every joint in my body so inflamed that it hurt to move or even cough. I had severe nausea and a burning fever that was rapidly rising. I couldn't move. For days I lay there unable to move.

A little voice inside began to grow louder and louder: "How are you taking care of yourself? What do you do for fun? Who are your friends? Where do you feel you belong? What is your sense of purpose and meaning in life?"

My visit with the doctor at the university health clinic was one of the most empty, cold, discouraging experiences of my life. I knew this was not the path to my healing this time.

My life has not been the same since that day. I left that doctor's office and turned to a warm, lively, very human group of alternative practitioners to support me in my healing process. I went deep within. I reconnected with my body, which still requires effort to this day. I began practicing yoga and meditation. I began moving my body more and doing those things that gave me joy as a young girl, such as ice skating and soccer. I moved to Montreal. I fell in love. I let go of a lot of old ways of thinking, old expectations, old agendas and behaviors that were no longer serving me. And I began doing work that felt like an expression of my true spirit. It felt meaningful because it helped other people.

It was an intense and radical healing crisis. It brought about intense and radical change. Every swollen joint, illness, and fever since then has been an opportunity for me to go within and ask some of those same questions.

Now, 12 years later, I am still practicing all of those things that brought me to wellness. It is a process, not a destination. My "to do list" toward well-being is not fixed. It changes every day as I change.

Books and other people have helped me on the way, and at times it has felt easier to think that someone else has the answer on a list in a book. It was easier to think that a healthcare practitioner or a remedy could do the healing for me, but I realized they can only help, support, or guide at most.

It is my intuition and body that knows what is right for me in each moment. I am the only one who can do the hard work of changing. Only I can give birth to my new self, over and over again. There is always a most healing choice. The trick is being quiet enough to hear and recognize that voice. If I lose the awareness or my life gets too full, sometimes it takes an incapacitating fever or flu to get my attention. Sometimes it only takes a big fight with my husband or a friend. Sometimes I notice it when I just feel really bad inside. Sometimes I just don't have the energy or desire to stay aware.

I've also found it valuable to view this process as a big healing bank account in the sky. Every good choice I make about my well being is like a deposit in the account. The truth is, the deposits add up over time. Getting too fixed and rigid or always feeling bad because I haven't done enough is constricting and cuts off the flow of life. It can also cut us off from other people.

I encourage you to wake up to your own inner voice. I offer only suggestions of what has worked for me.

PART TWO: BECOMING A PARENT

When I became a parent, I wanted to know more about helping myself and my family recover and heal from the many encounters with illnesses and injuries that naturally occur with young children. I was surprised at how terrifying it can be to care for a child with a high fever or a severe puncture wound. A trip to the doctor would often leave me with a prescription and not a lot of information about how to work with my child's condition. Our doctor seemed quick to fix and not really able to educate. The advice seemed fear-based and rigid, and his approach seemed unable to address the whole being.

When I turned to alternative medicine, I learned about homeopathy and herbs that brought comfort and healing. But the information often seemed to be opposed to mainstream medicine. I started feeling that resorting to antibiotics or Tylenol was considered failing. Red meat, dairy products, wheat, food additives, immunizations, disposable diapers, and global warming were seen as the culprits, but most at fault were conventional physicians. I personally believed that prescribed drugs had an important role as did prevention, homeopathy, and home therapies. I felt confused, frustrated, and placed in the middle to make difficult decisions.

When has a fever gone on too long? What are the early warning symptoms? What can I do at home to bring comfort and relief? How do I know if this herb or homeopathic remedy is really working? Am I giving the right remedy with so many symptoms to wade through to find the "right one"? How do I care for this wound or burn properly? Most of all, I wanted to know what to watch for and that we were safe and on the right track. That came slowly with education, time, and experience.

Over time and many trips to the doctor's office, I learned that with most common illnesses I was doing as much for myself or my child as they could do in the clinic--and sometimes more. I would come home with the prescription or drug and either use it or have it on hand in case we really needed it. Sometimes the antibiotics were critical and even life saving. But the more I learned about how to work with home therapies and a healing life-style, the less I needed to resort to pharmaceuticals. *The key was releasing myself from rigid dogmas and being flexible in the moment.*

HERE AND NOW

When an illness does arise, I now have a better sense of how to work with it before it gets too bad. Becoming experienced with home therapies and understanding the role of conventional medicine have been the keys.

Paying attention and working with my symptoms and my family's illnesses has been a healing in itself. It has required and inspired me to do the most difficult task of all: to care for my whole self every single day. It's an ever-changing process that takes practice, time, and effort. By doing this, I am living a much richer life. I have more physical vitality and fewer illnesses.

3

A HEALING LIFE-STYLE

SLEEP, REST, AND RHYTHM

One of the most difficult things for me to learn has been this business of rejuvenation. It is the challenge of our times because there is so much to do! Learning how to find the balance of doing and not doing, breathing in and breathing out, sleeping and waking has taken some effort and discipline. I'm still practicing.

Deep in our bodies, our organ functions possess a rhythm. Having a similar daily schedule of eating, sleeping , bathing, and working, helps our bodies stay in balance with these rhythms. Daily rhythmical repetition also strengthens the spirit, allowing us to be awake and alert as a vehicle for the human personality.

Enough sleep is one of the most important prerequisites to good health. Children especially need at least 12 hours of sleep each night to allow for full growth and development. Most adults in our culture also need more sleep than they are getting.

The process of going to sleep, with the slipping away of consciousness, occurs because the soul and spirit disengage themselves from the nervous system. We repeat this process several times each night and it is supplemented by longer or shorter episodes of rapid-eye-movement (REM) sleep during which an increase in the regenerative activity takes place.

I have found that letting go of the day with a short walk, a bath, or an artistic activity helps me prepare for sleep and I sleep more deeply. It is also nice to stand back and witness the events of the day in reverse order just before sleep. It helps to do this at a similar time every day. It's a way of slowly surrendering from the awake state of individual activity and transitioning into the regenerative sphere of sleep.

The seven-day rhythm, which is evident in the healing process of many infectious diseases (pneumonia, measles, typhoid) can also be supported by giving the days of the week their own emphasis. Certain things might be done only on Tuesdays, for instance, enabling the weekly rhythm to be imprinted more strongly. Weekly repetition strengthens the soul as the vehicle for thinking, feeling, and willing or doing.

Monthly repetition strengthens the forces which underlie growth and thinking. This has consequences for memory and recall capacity.

The yearly rhythm, in contrast, strengthens the physical body.[1]

Many of us already move in accord with these rhythms due to school calendars, work schedules, monthly menstrual cycles, and holidays, festivals, and birthdays celebrated at the same time each year. The shift comes when we bring our awareness and consciousness to these rhythms, deepening them in the smallest ways over time.

Start simply by bringing in a daily greeting here or a short bedtime ritual there. Then watch over time to notice the effects. Doing this has had a tremendously positive impact on my sense of well-being. I feel that it also helps children develop a strong physical constitution and creates in them a deep sense of security and belonging.

MOVEMENT

I so much prefer this word over the E word (Exercise). "Movement" has so much more potential and flexibility. It helps me keep more in touch with what my body needs in the moment. It can mean: scrubbing or sweeping a floor, dancing, going swimming at the lake, shoveling snow, playing frisbee, walking briskly to the store, practicing yoga, digging in the garden, mopping, working out at a gym, raking leaves with my family, or washing the car. I also have to add "taking a short rest or nap" to this list, because at times that is also what my body needs most.

It can also mean reading, meditating, writing a letter, making cookies, or playing the piano. The key, again, is flexibility, which leaves lots of opportunity to feel good about ourselves.

I could write volumes about the benefits of vigorous physical activity. However, by bringing your own awareness to this area of your life, the sense of well-being that you're likely to experience will speak for itself.

Movement is invigorating, life enhancing, strengthening, energizing, enlivening, rejuvenating, mood enhancing, cleansing, warmth generating, relaxing, and stress relieving. Every time I take my attention off of this area of my life, I don't feel as good, and I also feel less inclined to get up and do things. But somehow I keep finding my way back. The more I move, the better I feel, and the more motivated I am to keep moving. It's a process. The only choice we really ever have is to keep trying until it feels good.

NATURE

Spending time in nature, especially with children, is a vital part of our family's well being. It's refreshing, soothing, and it just plain feels good. We have tried to bring nature into our daily rhythm by having outdoor time at a similar time each morning. It helps us wake up our senses for the day ahead and seems to have a very positive effect on our moods.

Another way to bring nature into a weekly rhythm is by choosing a day of the week for a nature walk. Children love to gather natural objects: stones, pine cones, nuts and moss. Placing these objects artfully on a little table helps to bring nature indoors and keep us in touch with the rhythms of the seasons.

SING

Sing alone. Sing together.

I was surprised at how much inhibition I had about singing. We now sing at least once a day before a meal. I have noticed that if we come to the table in a less than harmonious way, or if I'm in a bad mood, it's almost as if I have to force myself to take hands and sing the song. But every time we take hands and sing, a feeling of "everything is going to be okay" comes over me, and it really changes the mood of the meal. It's better than Tums!

Singing together is good for the body and great for the soul. Are there places you could sneak it in? On the car ride to the store instead of a cassette tape? After a Sunday evening meal? At a holiday each year? Sing when and where you can, but do sing!

LET YOUR HOME FEED YOUR SOUL

In these hectic times, living simply is an art and an ongoing challenge. There is a constant pull to go, to do, to acquire, to accumulate. Keeping at bay the accumulation of stuff (clothes, papers, books, sheets, toys, magazines, dishes) seems to be one of our biggest challenges. When our home becomes chaotic and cluttered, it feels depleting. It takes too much time and energy to keep clean, and it eats away at our precious time for self-care.

Look around your house. Look at every object. Do you use it often? Does it add to your sense of well-being? Does it have sentimental value? Should it be stored away from the main living area? Does it have a permanent storage spot or home? Would someone else use it more than you? Can you let it go?

We recently went through a process in which the whole family went through every object in the house and agreed upon a place for it to live. We soon ran out of places. We let go of what there wasn't room for and stored some of the more precious objects in the basement. After we use something we try to put it back where it lives. Now that takes practice. We've also become rather vigilant about what comes into our home before it turns into another enormous pile of clutter.

This was a grueling process and I expect that we will have to do it again someday. But it has freed up an enormous amount of time and energy so that we can spend more time taking care of ourselves and doing fun things. It feels more peaceful and harmonious to be at home now. We have also cleared the way for new people and projects to come into our lives.

ACTIVITIES THAT GIVE JOY, MEANING, AND A SENSE OF PURPOSE

What activities do you get so lost in that you forget what time it is, and even forget to eat? What gives you joy? So much of living is the daily business of routines and obligations. We must consciously balance obligations with joy-filled activities.

The more I engage in joyful activity, the more meaning my life takes on. My life, my work, my contributions in the world feel more like an expression of who I am and less like a job. I feel more like I have a sense of purpose. I feel there really is a reason why I am here on this planet, and my contribution matters. Living in this way leads me to a deeper sense of being connected and belonging.

This sense of purpose is a very healing force. It is amplified for most people when that sense of purpose has a positive impact on other people's lives and the evolution of humanity.

NUTRITION

I saved this area until last because there tends to be too much emphasis upon food in our culture. "If we just had our diet down everything would be okay." It's only part of the picture.

Having said that, I confess I have been quite drawn to the subject and have been studying nutrition and experimenting with food for over 15 years: veganism, fruitarianism, vegetarianism, macrobiotics, and everything in between. What I have come to understand is that nutrition is far more than a study of fats, proteins, and carbohydrates. Eating well gives us the vital energy we need for personal and spiritual transformation. Without this vital energy we feel lethargic, unmotivated, cranky, and even sick.

For the last several years I have been eating rather well by using the "listen to your body" method. The danger I found was that when I was eating more sugar and processed foods, my body told me that it wanted more sugar and processed foods. So it's a balance of eating what feels right in the moment, but also having an overall framework of good guidelines and rhythms to keep our sense of taste trustworthy and on track.

I come from a long line of Mennonite farmers. Now those people cooked! Both men and women spent most of their waking hours growing, harvesting, preserving, cooking, and cleaning.

They came around the table together often. There were many traditions surrounding food. They often simmered and stirred a meal all day before it came to the table. The food had warmth and love in it. It was deeply satisfying and nourishing to the whole being. And they ate really fresh, unprocessed, whole foods.

Our society is moving farther and farther from preparing food at home and eating meals together. We want time to do other things. And we are rarely home all day to walk over to the stove and stir a simmering pot. The prepared foods and deli sections in supermarkets are the fastest growing area of the food industry. We are losing a tradition of cooking and eating together.

On the other hand, I am constantly impressed by the enormous amount of money, time, and energy it takes to eat well. Sometimes I have to choose to eat something less healthy because I'd rather go for a swim. Or our family would rather take a walk in the woods than spend the morning cooking and cleaning up after whole-grain blueberry pancakes. Where is the balance?

The following guidelines are our family's attempt to find balance and have the best of both worlds. The nutritional suggestions have helped me keep my taste buds on track. This way of eating has brought the greatest sense of satisfaction and nourishment on all levels.

Food Preparation Survival Guidelines

Share the Responsibility: In our family we have worked out a way that everyone takes on a portion of the cooking responsibilities, so they don't rest on one person. If family members can't cook, teach them. It's important. More important, it's fun to cook and clean up together. If you live alone, find another person with whom to share the cooking. It's a lot easier to cook twice as much while you're in the mode. It's also more motivating to cook for someone else while you do so for yourself. Take turns cooking with another family and share meals once or twice a week. Be creative. Keep trying.

Cook When You Cook: When you are planning a meal, think about how it can become lunch or supper for the next day. It's easier to make more and warm it up. This takes more planning but it drastically reduces the amount of cooking and cleaning time.

Cook With Joy: No matter how whole and organic our foods are, if they are prepared by someone who is rushing and feels overwhelmed and resentful, or eaten at a chaotic table, our meals can become almost like poison, despite our best intentions.

Experiment with the number of days a week that you choose to do the cooking until you find what feels like a balance to you. Then cook with all your heart. Think of how much you care about the loved ones who are going to eat this meal. Imagine how deeply it is going to feed them on all levels. Bring as much joy and love to the process as you can. See how this affects your experience of being nourished, both in cooking and eating.

Nourishing Traditional Food Selections

The following guidelines come from the book *Nourishing Traditions: The Cookbook that Challenges Politically Correct Nutrition and Diet Dictocrats* by Sally Fallon with Pat Connolly and Mary G. Enig. At first this book was quite challenging to read because it contradicts a lot of modern cultural messages. It brings a fresh look at nutrition based on thousands of years of anthropology, history, and comparative religion to the fascinating subject of ethnic and modern diets. It is also full of wonderfully nourishing recipes. It's one way! Try it for yourself and see if some of it feels right for you.

Carbohydrates: Whole-grain products (properly treated for the removal of phytates) such as sourdough and sprouted grain bread; soaked or sprouted cereal grains; soaked and fermented pulses and legumes including lentils, beans and chickpeas; sprouted or soaked seeds and nuts; fresh fruits and vegetables; fermented vegetables. Natural sweeteners such as honey, sucanat, and maple syrup.

Dairy: Raw, cultured organic dairy products such as yogurt, pima milk, kefir, and raw cheese.

Fats: Fresh butter and cream, preferably raw and cultured; animal fat; extra virgin olive oil; unrefined flax seed oil (in small amounts); coconut oil and other tropical oils.

Proteins: Fresh, organically raised meat including beef, lamb, chicken, turkey, and other fowl; organ meats from organically raised animals; seafood of all types from deep sea waters; fish eggs; fresh organic eggs; fermented soy products.

Beverages: Filtered, high-mineral water; lacto-fermented drinks made from grain or fruits; herb teas; meat and vegetable broths.

Condiments: Natural sea salt; raw vinegar; spices; and fresh herbs.[2]

BALANCE

The trick of course is in the juggling. It's the ability to be awake to as many of the various areas of your life as possible at once. For instance, in winter we put more emphasis on food. Summer may bring more attention to the outdoors and movement. The attention to rhythm helps us with this juggling process so that we don't get too far out of balance. But when we have lost the balance, we know it.

I have found Christmas to be a time when I am most likely to lose my balance. Long vacations, trips, and holidays also disrupt my daily routines and it takes extra attention to stay in touch with my body and sense of balance and well being. It seems I do much better with my simple weekly rhythm. At times I have found it helpful to make a little list and post it on the fridge to remind me of basic needs for self-care.

Remember, it's the heightened awareness and attention to these areas with small adjustments over time that lead to a deeper sense of well-being in body, emotions, mind, and spirit.

4

A Healing Approach to Illness

Illnesses and injuries can often mean that some part of our being is out of balance. Physical symptoms can sometimes be preceded by an emotional or mental upset. Ongoing strain in the way we bring ourselves to a certain relationship may lead to a physical breakdown. We are whole beings with interconnected parts. Physical illness is an opportunity to reflect, to pull back from the busyness of our everyday lives and check in. A healing crisis is ultimately an opportunity to grow.

THE MEANING OF ILLNESS

When illnesses become chronic or symptom patterns continue to repeat themselves, questions can arise. Why won't this dreaded symptom just go away? Why me? Why does it always seem to flare up under certain circumstances? These questions can ultimately lead us to wonder about a deeper meaning behind our condition.

I wonder. . . could it be related to a behavior or belief or relationship dynamic? What was happening in your life when the symptoms began? Do the symptoms have a pattern? Was there a particularly physical or emotional trauma experienced at the onset of the symptoms? Are you happy in your relationships, your job? What is going on in your life right now?

For many people physical symptoms can carry a deep memory or message about a deeper need for balance and healing in our emotional, mental, or spiritual lives. Illness provides us an opportunity to go inward and pay attention to that delicate balance. It can invite us to wake up to new parts of ourselves. Making a change in the dynamics of a relationship, reassessing or clearing an old belief pattern that is no longer serving us-- these are some of the ways we can free up stuck energy and make room for more joy, creativity, vitality, and sense of purpose in our lives.

The healing process begins by having the courage to ask the questions, then taking time to go within to listen and pay attention. Take a minute to bring all your attention to a particular part of your body or a painful symptom. Breath into it. What do you notice? If you stay there long enough does it change? See if this approach works for you.

If you are inclined to look a bit deeper, the healing process can be accelerated with the support of a practitioner. There are many body-mind-spirit modalities that can offer this approach. To mention two, both Process Work and Process Acupressure were designed to facilitate holistic healing and bring understanding and meaning to illness. Process Work, founded by Arnold Mindel, helps you to uncover what is behind symptoms and gain a deeper insight into the self. Process Acupressure, originated by Aminah Raheem, combines process work with a hands-on approach of holding acupressure points to promote healing and responsibility for one's own wellness.

Working in these ways has helped me get to the core meaning of symptom patterns and connect with a deep sense of inner guidance. I have also worked out emotional and relational patterns that were causing me a great deal of pain. As a result, I feel a greater sense of purpose, balance, and joy in my everyday life . I am also more capable of working things out on my own when difficulties arise. Physical symptoms have also resolved themselves as a by product of this process.

Regardless of the chosen therapy, the effectiveness largely depends on your level of trust in the practitioner. Trust your instincts. It is best to work with someone who is willing to help you follow your own process and go to a deep level of guidance within. Agendas, advice, interpretation and analysis are usually not extremely helpful when working in this way. Always try to be clear about what your intentions are. [3] (See "Personal and Spiritual Transformation" in the Further Reading section of the appendix.)

ILLNESS AND HEALING

Dr. Philip Incao, an internationally recognized anthroposophical physician, states:

"Healing is our being's attempt to grow and restore balance in our lives. It is also our physical body's attempt to restore well-being and vitality. We are always exposed to and often harbor germs, and yet we only occasionally get sick. Why do we get sick when we do?

"Most common illnesses are inflammations. 'Infection' is the wrong word for them because it suggests that we get sick because germs invade us. This is misleading.

"In order to stay healthy we must keep an inner balance in body and soul while at the same time growing and changing from birth to death. We also remodel and renew our bodies many times along the way. Every remodeling job requires some demolition, a breaking down of part of our inherited body structure in order to rebuild it better. This breaking down of old cells and tissues results in debris that must be cleared before the body can rebuild itself.

"It is the immune system which does the breaking down by creating fever and inflammation to destroy and digest foreign or outworn bodily material. It is the immune system which cleans up the digested material and debris by pushing it out of the body. Debris that remains in the body may act like a poison or may cause allergies or repeated inflammations later on. Skin rashes, discharges, or mucus or pus are signs that our immune systems are actively working.

"Most colds, sore throats, and earaches are a healing crisis and a cleansing process, making way for our renewed bodies and our new selves."[4]

Hering's Law of Cure:

Dr. Constantine Hering, formulated principles that govern the direction of a cure. He stated:

- Cure takes place from within outwards, meaning that most vital organs will get better first. So the brain, lungs, heart, liver, and kidneys will improve before the gut, muscles, joints or skin.

- Cure takes place from above to below; for example, psoriasis should clear up first on the head followed by the hands.
- Cure takes place in reverse order to the onset of symptoms. If a child has a history of eczema but presents with asthma, as the asthma is cured, the eczema should return before healing for good.[5]

THE VALUE OF FEVER

Hippocrates said, "Fever is half the striving of the organism against disease. It purifies the body like fire."

Dr. Incao suggests that, "Fever is the ultimate assistant in this remodeling project. Viruses and bacteria in us grow faster when the body temperature is lower, and they are destroyed faster by the body's immune system when the body temperature is higher."[6]

"Fever also stimulates and trains immunological resistance in the body. It also stimulates and trains thermo-regulation and consequently, blood circulation in all the organs.

Anyone who takes human development into account when treating an illness will avoid indiscriminate use of fever-suppressing drugs, just as they will be careful not to exclude their use on principle. Every case of a high temperature needs to be cared for with regard to the person's unique needs and capabilities. One person may 'need' a temperature to increase the activity of the metabolism and immune system and allow it to 'work at' the physical constitution. But another may need protection from being weakened by an excessive febrile reaction."[7] (See "Fever" in Section Six for more practical information on home care.)

A HEALING PRESENCE

The importance of a calm, centered, loving presence is invaluable to the healing process. It is particularly significant in the face of a first aid crisis, when it is important to stay grounded and make fast decisions. When faced with the sudden onset of an illness or an injury, stop and take a few deep breaths. What are your questions? How can you quickly rule out a medical emergency? Do you have a system in place to help you make clear decisions in the moment? Do you have access to information that allows you to know the parameters of safety? Do you have any healing substances at home that could help in this situation? Do you have ready access to a reference that reminds you exactly how to use them?

This guide and other reference materials may be very helpful. However, part of the calm, confident, loving presence you need just comes with experience over time. Eventually you become more familiar with how to work with certain sets of symptoms.

When an unfamiliar illness pops up, or an illness has gone on longer than usual, fear can enter the picture. The ill person immediately senses this, and it can be like a poison to the healing process if it goes too long without being noticed. When you sense this fear, it's just a sign that you have reached the edge of your comfort zone. It's good. It's natural. Go back to square one with your questions and decision-making process until you feel like you're on the right track again. Most important, pay close attention to this voice. You may actually need to seek more medical attention.

Jackson's Story

My son Jackson, at three years old, had a history of allergies and eczema. He had episodes of becoming pale, with loss of appetite, weakness, and an immediate need to sleep. Usually by morning he was fine.

One night he developed these symptoms with the addition of a high fever. He complained of a stiff neck and a sore back and headache. He showed no signs of meningitis. These symptoms persisted for four or five days. The fever would come and go and at times would be very high. He became less and less interested in food and water. He became more glassy eyed, lethargic, and withdrawn. He did not seem himself at all, and this was the most disturbing part. At one point he picked up a bit and began to show signs of hunger and thirst.

By the sixth day his fever was high again and he seemed farther and farther away. We consulted our doctor and he found no signs of an underlying infection.

By day seven his fever was going down, but he showed signs of dehydration. At that point he also began breathing through his nose for the first time in a year. And, amazingly, his skin cleared up. That day we visited the doctor again. He suggested that our son be brought back that evening to the ER for intravenous fluids. Jackson was refusing to drink and really starting to fade. I was exhausted. I was scared and worried.

I knew I only had a few hours before we went to the ER. When I got home I contacted our family anthroposophical physician, who gave me a few suggestions. I felt empowered to at least try them in the little time remaining. I gathered dandelions from the yard and brewed a batch for a poultice for his liver. I prepared lemon for leg compresses. Chamomile tea was brewed, which was to be given rectally (the orifice of last resort to be used as a place fluids can be absorbed). An anthroposophical remedy was suggested. All of these measures were to help stimulate his life forces and help "bring him back."

I remember walking into his room with a tray full of steaming pots of herbs and compresses. I felt very strong and optimistic. "Jackson, you're coming back," I asserted rather confidently as I approached him. I offered him a remedy with a drink of water and he actually took a sip of water without any resistance, which seemed as if it hadn't happened in days. On some level he was agreeing with me that it was, in fact, time to come back.

As I applied the bitter dandelion compress to his liver he fell fast asleep. He retained the brewed chamomile enema, and I applied lemon to his legs. He rested more soundly than he had for a very long time.

When he woke up he seemed a little more willing to drink. I repeated the regimen. He slept again. And again he improved on waking. By that evening he had more color in his cheeks and was less glassy eyed. I finally could sense his presence again. From that point he continued to improve.

This was an extreme example of walking the fine line between home therapies and mainstream medicine. The key in this situation was having the support of a trusted healthcare provider when we felt we couldn't go on. At the same time we were empowered to continue by knowing the symptoms we could watch for that would indicate a need for further medical care. In this case we were able to avoid a potentially traumatic trip to the emergency room for intravenous fluids.

In addition, Jackson's allergies and eczema have continued to improve dramatically. The healing plants, combined with the fever, helped him to transform himself at a very deep level. He also seemed much more grown up after he fully recovered.

Finally, this experience had a profound effect on Jackson's and my relationship. We went through something very intense and scary together. We learned a way of negotiating and relating to each other that has set a very positive precedent as other illnesses have come and gone. Sitting together in the silence of that experience helped deepen our relationship and understanding of each other in a way that is still beyond words.

THE WELL-BEING OF THE CAREGIVER

Supporting someone through an illness or healing crisis can take an enormous amount of energy and stamina. One person's well-being should not be at the expense of another's. The caregiver must assess his or her own internal resources before choosing to engage in that role and again at points during the entire healing process. Family and friends can also be called upon for support. The intention of the caregiver must be to help the ill person tap into his or her own healing resources to regain strength and vitality. Well-being is promoted by doing only what is necessary and not doing for the patient the things they can do for themselves. Here's a checklist for your self -care:

1) Physical: Pay attention to your own needs for rest, good nutrition, fluids, and fresh air. Pause frequently to check in with your body.

2) Emotional: Have an emotional support system in place if possible. When you feel yourself becoming afraid, go back to square one and make sure you're on the right track or call on a trusted friend or healthcare provider for feedback and consultation.

3) Psychological: Adequate rest will help you stay mentally alert and balanced. Be flexible. Either/or's can lead to discouragement. Remember, you can feel good about the fact that you are choosing as many supportive, life-enhancing tools as possible, and take care of your self.

4) Spiritual: Draw upon prayer, meditation, visualization, affirmations, and healing thoughts.

Is there meaning in illness? Does every little symptom require so much attention and analysis? Probably not! By simply entertaining the question, or even bringing your awareness to a symptom, you open yourself to new healing potential. This section of the guide simply provides a philosophy of healing or way to imagine illnesses and imbalances. It is one of the many ways. While sailing the stormy waters of a health crisis, it helps to have a philosophical foundation. It will anchor you so that you can open yourself to new possibilities as you begin choosing and integrating the various paths of care.

5

CHOOSING A PATH OF CARE

When illnesses and imbalances occur, questions can often arise. Should I see a doctor right away? What can he or she do for me? When should I use herbs, natural medicines, and home therapies? What can I do on my own at home to promote healing? This section is like a road map that will help you navigate through these questions and show you that all of these options are available to you at any point in the healing process.

The first path empowers you and teaches you how to strengthen your own inner healing forces. Use these care-giving measures as much as you can. You will be much more likely to achieve results with the following paths if these care-giving measures are in place.

The second path shows how natural medicines and home therapies can also support the healing process. These substances can help alleviate symptoms and bring balance to the entire system. Though the results can be immediate, this path typically offers a more long-term benefit. Over time you may notice that the symptoms become less severe when they show up, and you and your body have become smarter and stronger in finding your way back to health.

Finally, the third path ties in the important role of conventional medicine. Prescribed drug therapy can be extremely effective in quickly relieving severe and life-threatening symptoms. This path can help to stabilize a condition so that you have the peace of mind and the energy to continue working with paths one and two.

These paths are mutually inclusive. With the support of a healthcare provider you can move between them, depending on the circumstance.

PATH ONE: SUPPORTING THE HEALING PROCESS

Our body's innate healing powers have the ability to overcome most imbalances and common illnesses. Caring for the whole person through proper nutrition, fluids, warmth, rest, and care of the senses are the most critical ways to address any illness. The early use of these care-giving measures enhances the patient's opportunity to come out of the illness stronger, with more antibodies and white blood cells to reduce the likelihood of recurrence. Even if remedies, antibiotics, or other pharmaceuticals are taken, these principles of care are still the key to supporting a deeper healing and must be continued until well-being is reestablished. Healing requires us to have the courage to step back from the busyness of life and care for ourselves and our loved ones. Overcoming an illness in this way can then lead to new-found personal and spiritual strength and development.

CARING FOR THE SENSES

A sick person's senses are often more susceptible to outside impressions. Creating a calm, peaceful mood in the room will allow more attention and life energy to go toward the healing process. In general, human sounds are much more soothing than electronic ones. Could this be an opportunity to turn off the radio and television?

Take a minute to really look around and listen. If the person is confined to a bed, what will they be looking at and listening to all day? Could the space use some tidying? Does he or she like to have some flowers on a table or a few familiar objects in view? Is there a table near the bed for a glass of fresh water and a place to set a bowl? Does the patient need his or her hands and face washed? Is the room well ventilated? Are the lights too bright? Is there a way to make the room more soundproof? Are the linens clean?

Attention to this kind of detail will allow the person to get right to the healing process without a lot of distraction.

NUTRITION

When someone is coming down with a cold or fever the sick person often loses his or her appetite. This is the body's way of turning its life forces toward healing. When the body is trying to eliminate toxic substances, it helps if it doesn't have to digest a lot of food at the same time. Therefore, the general rule is to cut back on or avoid protein foods during an acute febrile illness. Foods high in protein are: meat, eggs, dairy, nuts, fish, and legumes. The sick person's diet should largely consist of broths, soups, herb teas, and room-temperature fruit juices. Fruit, cooked vegetables, grains, and light breads are also suitable.

Another general rule: when sick, eating less is better than eating more. If the ill person is not hungry, then he or she is better off not eating.

The return of appetite is a sign of getting over the illness. But those first meals after the fever is gone should be light ones. Reintroduce the restricted food gradually and carefully. [8]

FLUIDS

It is so important to drink copious quantities of fluid during an illness, especially if there is a fever. Dehydration can develop very quickly with a fever, especially with young children and older people. Once dehydration sets in, the thought of drinking actually becomes nauseating. Eventually, drinking even a small amount can result in vomiting.

Dr. Thomas Cowan suggests: "Dehydration can lead to prolongation of fever and further nausea, and it can actually inhibit or delay the healing process. Dehydrated people look sick; they are weak and pale with sunken eyes and dry mouth, and they have decreased urine production. (See "Dehydration" in Section Six for more information on home care.)

"Warm teas and broths are best to nourish and prevent dehydration. Here are some suggestions for preparing broths:

"Chicken broth: sauté onions, carrots and celery in a small amount of butter; then add a whole, naturally-raised chicken, water, and sea salt. Bring to a boil and simmer for several hours. Strain and serve warm.

"Vegetable broth: gently cook some onions in butter or olive oil. Add fresh vegetables, sea salt and garlic to your liking. Bring to a boil and simmer for several hours. Strain and serve warm.

"In the beginning it is best to drink only broth. As the appetite and vitality return, begin adding in vegetables and then grains."[9]

BATHS

Hydrotherapy is highly effective for acute illnesses. Baths are not only soothing and relaxing, but they can also aid in elimination through our largest sense organ, the skin. Healing substances can also be added to the bath water to be absorbed through the skin. Warm baths can also aid in enhancing our bodily warmth. Alternating warm and cold temperature can stimulate the vascular system and aid in the healing process. Dr. Cowan suggests the following in his patient handout:

"At the onset of a cold, flu, or fever, try the following*:

1) Drink 8 oz. of hot herbal tea (if possible include Elder flower and Peppermint). These teas are all good in helping induce a sweat.

2) Get into a very hot bath for 15 minutes or so.

3) For one minute get into a very cold shower.

4) Immediately wrap up in a towel, blanket, or warm clothes and get into a bed with a warmed hot-water bottle.

5) Stay in bed for as long as there is any dizziness or feeling of weakness.

6) Continue to drink plenty of water, tea and broth.

This should make you sweat profusely. It is best to have someone assist you, since a vague sense of dizziness will often occur.

*This method DOES NOT APPLY if the temperature is over 101 degrees F., or to children under 10, the elderly, pregnant women, or those in otherwise poor general health.[10]

REST

SLEEP IS THE BEST HEALER! Never wake up the ill person to give a remedy or take a temperature.

WARMTH

A normal body temperature is 98.6 degrees F. or slightly higher. A subnormal temperature indicates that not enough warmth is being produced by the body. Viruses and bacteria grow faster when the body temperature is lower, and they are destroyed faster by the body's immune system when the body temperature is higher.

When a person has a fever, it is important to stay comfortably warm with as many layers of cotton and wool as tolerable. The body, in its wisdom, wants and needs to be hot in order to burn out the illness.[11]

TOUCH AND MASSAGE

Massage, with the aid of a pleasant-smelling or aromatic oil, can bring great comfort to someone who is sick. It can bring circulation and relief to aching lower back muscles. It also helps bring a general sense of well-being and relaxation that might allow a deeper rest or sleep to follow.

It is helpful if the experience is quieting. Slow, gentle, rhythmic movements will bring the greatest sense of peace and well-being. It is also good to wrap the person up warmly or swaddle the body after the massage to stimulate a heat reaction.

HEALING OBJECTS

In our family's healing kit there is a little crystal. On the shelf beside the kit we have set a wooden healing bowl and cloth. When someone gets a scrape or bump, we fill the bowl with warm water and sometimes add a drop or two of lavender oil to soak the injured part. The crystal goes on the table by the bed or in the feverish hand.

These sacred objects come out only during times of healing. They help us create a special place, set apart from the routine of daily life, to honor the healing process. These special objects can send deep signals to that healing part of us that we don't encounter every day.

PATH TWO: HOME THERAPIES

The remedies and natural medicines covered in this guide are derived from plants and minerals as they occur in nature. They are prepared to capture the healing essence of the entire organism. Each plant and mineral carries specific healing properties that can help provide a picture of wholeness to our bodies when they become out of balance. In fact, it has been said that every plant on earth represents an illness in humans. Meaning, the essence of each plant carries energy or qualities of corresponding illnesses.

When we are really sick we can feel that our true self or inner being is at the mercy of our body or the illness. When we take a plant remedy and introduce the proper corresponding quality, it permits our true being to engage in the healing process.

On a purely physical level, plants and minerals can also be very effective in supporting the innate healing process in its effort to cleanse, rebuild, and regenerate new, healthy tissue.

Remedies and natural medicines can be helpful when the person is not bouncing back easily on his or her own or when it seems important to care for a pattern of symptoms or a weakened constitution. Depending on the situation or your style of treatment they can also be taken at the onset of symptoms to "nip it in the bud," so to speak. They can also be used in combination with prescribed drug therapy to help the person cleanse and regain strength after a prolonged illness.

Remember that the healing influence of plants and minerals may take more effort and time than many of us are used to in our quick-fix culture. The timing is slower. The process can sometimes feel like two steps forward and one step back. Be prepared to have persistence, patience, and a longer-term vision of the healing process.

The following is a deeper look at how plants and minerals bring a healing effect to the body. It is taken from *Caring for the Sick at Home* by Bentheim.

THE BODY

In a simplified way, the body can be seen as having three major systems that need to be in balance to sustain harmony and well-being. Two of the systems are polar opposites with the third being the mediator. They are the nervous system, the metabolic digestive system, and the rhythmic system.

> **The nervous system** or the upper pole represents our conscious ability to think and perceive. This system allows us to create new thoughts and ideas.

It is centered in our hard head, which is the coolest part of our body. This system of nerves runs throughout our entire body. Cells from the nervous system die very quickly and do not readily regenerate themselves. They are always close to death and are exquisitely sensitive to lack of oxygen and blood. To see a stroke victim, for example, shows us muscles that are no longer stimulated by living nerves. The lens of the eye and ear drum are made of nearly dead, hardened matter much like a quartz crystal.

> **The metabolic/digestive system** is the lower pole and allows us to regenerate and to act. This system allows us to regenerate and create new living cells.

It is centered in our belly and limbs. It is here that we humans generate warmth and transform food into usable energy that allows us to move our limbs. The reproductive organs also live in this area and represent our greatest potential for regeneration. The liver and spleen are able to regenerate if part of them is removed.

These processes are done unconsciously. The organs in this system possess cells with regenerative forces that contrast sharply with the cells of the nervous system. The working of the metabolic system can be seen in the inflammatory process of producing red, hot, tender and swollen tissue. Hot, soft and alive. Here again in contrast to the nervous system.

The rhythmic system is the mediator and is the center of respiration and rhythm. It is where our breath, blood flow, and heartbeat originate.

The heart is the central point for the blood that comes down from the head and up from the belly. The blood is enlivened through breathing oxygen in the lungs and given back again to each respective pole. The heart beats unconsciously, much like the other activities of the lower pole. The lungs breathe with more conscious awareness and thus are more related to the nerve/sense pole.

The blood is the mode of transportation for the body's healing army, in that the blood carries antibodies, other proteins, and white blood cells. The immune system is where we most deeply distinguish what is foreign from what is "self." "What is me? What is not me? What is my true identity?" In a way, the true self or spirit can be thought of as being carried in the blood.

Therefore, during an illness, supporting the rhythmic system with warmth and nourishment is critical for empowering the immune system to do its job. In doing so, you are supporting and empowering your "self."

Illness, simply put, begins when the balance is tipped too much toward one pole or the other. For instance, an ear infection is an inflammation, a warmth process which belongs in the belly but is now invading the upper pole or nervous system. Gallstones in the belly represent a hardening process that belongs to the upper pole but has traveled down to the lower pole due to an imbalance.

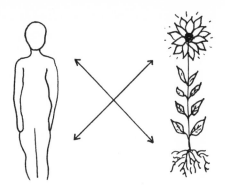

Figure 1.

PLANTS

By observing the physical nature and essence of the plant, we can see the same three processes that we saw at work in the human body's three major systems. In a way the plant can be seen as an upside-down human, as is shown in Figure 1.

The root or lower pole is the center of the sensory system or "nervous system" of the plant, and it possesses nodes of cells that sense gravity. Roots live in the depths of the cold, hard earth, where they transport the dead or unenlivened minerals. Visually roots resemble the branching network of nerves in the human body.

The flower or upper pole is closest to the sun and is where the warmth enters the plant. It is also where the plant holds the seed and the regenerative possibilities of new life.

The leaf is the mediator. It is where the plant breathes, exchanging oxygen and carbon dioxide much like the lung does.

Upon closer observation, we can see that many plants can also have a one-sided nature, manifesting either an extensive root, flower, or leaf development. Onion, for example, has a root system that is more developed than the leaves and flowers. These strengths serve as an operating "example" for the human organism when given as remedy. They provide a picture of wholeness that supports the body's innate ability to heal and regain vitality and energy. They can also help promote the cleansing process.

MINERALS

Minerals also have an important healing impact and work most deeply in the realm of the physical body. In order to gain more understanding of the healing properties of mineral and metal remedies, we must pay more attention to their essential nature and function than their physical appearance.

Silica, for example, in its natural form is hard, crystalline, and clear. Light easily penetrates its crystals. It can also be easily penetrated by tones, as when a glass is shattered by a high note. Silica's nature is much like our nervous system in its ability to perceive and carry light and sound. In Silicon Valley it is highly valued for its use in storing and transmitting information in computer chips.

In humans, silica is highly concentrated in the nervous system and sensory organs (brain tissue, skin, eyes and eardrums). As a remedy one can see how and why it brings clarity, structure, and strength to these nerve-sense organs.

Iron is a metal that eagerly binds to water and oxygen, as seen in its ability to rust easily. In our bodies, it is the carrier of oxygen in the form of hemoglobin. Without this crucial metal to carry it, oxygen would not be able to find its way to the brain and bring consciousness and mental clarity to the human being. Oxygen also brings energy to cells, lending vital and regenerative forces to the body's innate healing processes.[12]

THE HEALING RELATIONSHIP BETWEEN THE BODY, PLANTS, AND MINERALS

We can now begin to imagine the body's intimate connection to the plant and mineral world. In the examples below, it is crucial to focus on the qualitative or symbolic nature of the relationships.

Suppose that the upper pole or the nervous/sensory system processes have been weakened in a person. Maybe there is an inflammation causing excessive warmth in the head region, where the conditions are normally cool. Consequently, mental clarity and perception are diminished. The principles outlined above show that a healthier balance may be restored by introducing a plant with a one-sided nature visibly centered in the lower pole or root.

For example, in the case of an ear infection, the warmth process has moved into the head, where it should be cool. The onion, with its one-sided nature in the root or lower pole, helps guide the body back to balance. On a practical level, an onion compress can also help to draw out the infection and relieve pain.

In contrast, the flowers and seeds of the plant tend to affect the metabolic or digestive system and the limbs, while plants whose strength and one-sided nature lie in the leaf have a healing and balancing effect on the rhythmic system in the heart and lung region.

Minerals bring more specific functions to the processes or area of illness. The goal in using a mineral therapeutically is to prepare the substance so that it is directed to a specific bodily or organ function.[13] As we discuss the natural medicines more specifically in Section Eight, these patterns and relationships should become even clearer.

The following is a list of the specific kinds of home therapies covered in this guide in Section Eight.

Homeopathy and Anthroposophical Remedies

Homeopathy, as developed by Dr. Samuel Hahnemann, uses diluted plant and mineral substances to stimulate the body's natural defenses. The homeopathic remedies are prepared through a process called "potentization," which involves repetitively diluting and forcefully agitating the substance until the toxic effects have disappeared and the essence of the substance is activated in the solution.

Homeopathy is founded on Hahnemann's principle of "like cures like." For example, if a person ingests willow bark, he or she may develop hectic fevers. Malaria can also cause hectic fevers. Taking a potentized form of willow bark can help cure the symptoms associated with malaria.[14]

Anthroposophical remedies also use plant and mineral substances and also take advantage of the principle of "potentization."

Anthroposophical remedies are uniquely prepared based on an understanding of the relationship between the body and the upside-down plant as described above (see Fig. 1). The remedies direct healing properties to specific bodily functions according to the specialized ways in which they are prepared.

For instance, a warming process, such as heating, boiling, or burning, can be used which prepares the remedy to work in the metabolic system. A cooling process can be used to direct the remedy to the nervous system. A rhythmic process may be applied by exposing the remedy to the morning and evening sun for several days. This gives forces to the substances that protect them from deterioration. This rhythmic process ultimately prepares the remedy to be active in the rhythmic system.

Finally, anthroposophical remedies are prepared with the belief that imbuing the medicines with the highest healing intentions and human care will bring the greatest benefit.

Essential Oils

Healing oils are found in all parts of the plant and provide their aroma. These essences contain the living element, often referred to as the "soul" of the plant, which provides each plant with its own life force, its own energies and healing powers.

They can be used by placing a few drops on a cold compress for first aid needs (see lavender). They can also be used in humidifiers and baths (see eucalyptus).

Healing Foods

The therapeutic qualities of natural foods can have a direct effect on the body through the skin. They can be used in baths, poultices, and compresses (see onion, lemon, cottage cheese).

External Applications

External applications are herbal preparations applied as compresses, poultices, and wraps. Natural fibers are soaked in healing substances and then wrapped around the body or applied to specific parts that need healing. They can be hot or cold, depending on the desired effect.

The materials used for compresses and poultices should always be made of natural fibers such as wool, silk, cotton, linen, or flannel. These materials allow a breathing or interaction to take place between the curative quality of the substance and the body's reaction to it. The skin is the most important organ in this activity. Synthetic fibers are impermeable and allow little air to flow through them and thus are to be avoided if possible.

On a more human note, external applications help us work with the warmth element. How we direct, redirect, create, and release warmth is what heals us. Wraps provide a medium for warmth. Mary Charmichael writes: "A very sick friend once told me that wraps made her feel secure and guarded as though she was in the wings of angels. Imagine someone creating a cocoon for you to rest and heal in. Wraps are about ensouling a person who needs time off from a busy world; time to work through some of the coldness of life, or perhaps time to catch up and move on as they mold their individual lives".[15]

Your family may want to create a time when you treat each other to a wrap or compress when you are not ill. Now there's an idea!

Substance Baths

The water element brings life and is a tremendous mediating substance in the healing process. In a substance bath something is added to the water in order to surround the whole person with its healing properties. These substances can be teas, essential oils, or minerals, as well as foods (see chamomile, lemon, lavender, eucalyptus).

Inhalations

Inhalations use the healing properties of the essential oils usually derived from the flowers of the plant. The healing oils become airborne with the steam from boiling water or a room vaporizer. They are most commonly used to promote healing from colds, coughs, sinus infection or other respiratory conditions (see chamomile and eucalyptus).

Teas

Teas are prepared to drink or to be used as a compress or wrap. Flowers are to be covered with boiling water and left to steep for one minute. Leaves are steeped two to three minutes. Stalks, roots, and bark are covered with cold, fresh water, boiled for five minutes, and left to steep for five minutes. Strain and use as recommended.

Enemas

An enema with brewed chamomile can be given as a laxative or to help soothe and heal the irritated lining of the lower intestine. The colon's main job is to absorb fluids and turn loose stool into formed stool. Retention enemas can take advantage of this absorptive process to rehydrate the body through the colon.

Enema bags and prepackaged enema kits can be purchased from the drug store. If you buy the kit, simply empty out the solution, wash the bottle with hot soapy water, rinse very thoroughly, and fill with brewed chamomile at room-temperature. The bottles are prelubricated and disposable.

Three things to remember about administering enemas are: 1) make sure the tip is well lubricated, 2) insert it very slowly, letting the natural direction of the rectum guide you and 3) always squirt a few drops of the water or brewed chamomile on the inside of your wrist to ensure a comfortable temperature before you begin. If you have other questions or concerns about administering an enema, consult a healthcare provider for further instruction.

PATH THREE:

COMMONLY PRESCRIBED DRUG THERAPY

Prescribed drugs have a valuable role in the healing process. There are advantages and disadvantages to their use and they are sometimes overused. What's important is to know how and when to use them.

ADVANTAGES

Most drugs are synthetically generated compounds. Others are derived by isolating specific plant molecules. They are often designed to relieve or completely stop symptoms by altering very specific cellular activity and organ function. They are most effective in treating severe symptoms and life-threatening illness.

They can also quickly relieve minor symptoms like a runny nose. Pseudoephedrine, for instance, causes the blood vessels in the lining of the nose and sinuses to constrict, leading to a decrease in the production of mucus.

Prescribed drugs can also be valuable for prolonged, milder illnesses when both the caregiver and the patient need relief. Sometimes having the drug on hand can provide peace of mind or avoid a trip out in the middle of the night.

DISADVANTAGES

The main disadvantages of prescribed drug therapy are the side effects. Unfortunately, these compounds cannot always differentiate the cells or proteins in one area from another. Pseudoephedrine, for instance, cannot tell the difference between the blood vessels in the nose and in the heart. So, when taken, it can also cause the heart rate and blood pressure to increase in those who take it. Antibiotics, designed to destroy unwanted bacteria, can also harm necessary, healthy flora or bacteria in the vagina and colon, leading to yeast infection and diarrhea.

True healing is often absent from a purely drug-centered approach. Just because the symptom has been alleviated, it does not necessarily mean that healing has occurred. In fact, repeatedly stopping symptoms without caring for the whole being can lead to more severe symptoms or relapses. It has recently been recognized by conventional medicine that indiscriminate use of antibiotics for virally related sore throats often leads to the development of more frequent sore throats and relapses of the same![16]

COMPLETING THE HEALING

Once the symptoms have been alleviated, it is so tempting to jump back into our busy lives and stop taking care of ourselves. This can create a very long, drawn-out recovery process with prolonged lowered resistance and low energy. If a secondary illness or relapse occurs in this state, it is usually much worse the second time around.

After pharmaceutical treatment, the underlying causes of the symptom must still be healed. This is done first and foremost by supporting the innate healing process. With ongoing attention to ample rest, warmth, fluids, and care of the senses, the body will naturally clear out dead cells and rebuild new vital tissue. Remedies can also be used to support this process.

For instance, when antibiotics are used to treat bronchitis, the cough can often persist after they have destroyed the bacteria. Inhalations can help the body slough off or rid itself of the dead tissue in the lungs. Echinacea can help strengthen the immune system and kill bacteria. Baths and chest rubs can continue to bring warmth to the area and promote healing. Other remedies can be taken to help the body regenerate vital new lung cells.

It is very helpful to have a physician or healthcare provider whom you trust who also has knowledge of both mainstream medicine and home therapies, or who is at least supportive of your style of healing at home.

Obviously prescribed drugs must be administered with extreme care under the care of a physician or healthcare provider.

A LESSON IN DEPLETION (KIDNEY INFECTION)

Stinging, burning, urgent urination. I have had bladder infections before, but this one came on fast. I immediately started drinking plenty of water and tried to take a nap. However, that evening I had guests arriving from out of town, so I got up and did a lot of work around the house. When I look back, I can remember feeling that I was pushing my body too hard, but unfortunately that voice was overridden.

The next morning, I had blood in my urine and was in a lot of pain. I resolved to care for myself and began doing chamomile steams, fluids, rest, and warm abdominal compresses. I also called my physician and filled a prescription for an antibiotic. I kept the antibiotic on hand, but I wanted to wait a little longer to see if there were any signs of healing. Something told me that I had waited too long to begin more active self-care.

In the middle of the night I felt a shift . . . for the worse. I started to feel a very deep ache around my middle back and kidney region. I remember telling my husband that something really wrong was happening. It was a very dark night.

I looked at the antibiotic on the table, and I sensed that its time had come. But as I went to take it, I had an unexpected thought: "I wonder if it's safe to take this if I'm pregnant?" I wasn't trying to conceive nor was I even vaguely suspicious that I might be pregnant, but I followed my instinct.

The physician overseeing my care confirmed that Bactrim was contraindicated during pregnancy. I chose not to take a risk and began taking a more appropriate antibiotic. It was very strong and geared toward the developing kidney infection.

Then I got sick. Really sick. Until then I really didn't even know where my kidneys were. Now they were screaming. I was bedridden for two or three days in a tremendous amount of pain. I have never felt that close to darkness or dying.

I immediately called my anthroposophic physician to find a way to support the healing process while continuing to take the antibiotic. Based on our conversation, I did the following things several times a day: I applied ointments to the skin surrounding my kidneys and bladder to bring warmth and regenerative forces. I took remedies to help my body regain balance and soothe the inflammation. By alternately ingesting alkaline and acidic substances, I helped to create an unfavorable environment for the bacteria in my urinary tract. Finally, warm chamomile abdominal compresses brought great comfort and relief.

These measures sustained me. To my surprise, I never developed a fever and there was no need for hospitalization. Both of these typically occur with severe kidney infection.

As I worked through this illness I also had quite a dialogue with myself. This underlying sense of deep depletion kept haunting me. Why was I so depleted? The answers were not far behind. I saw very clearly how, for several years, I had been overextending myself in two important relationships. I saw how I was overriding the small voice that knew where the balance was. I saw how I needed to change.

It's been eight months since I recovered from that kidney infection. I can still feel my right kidney. It gently reminds me when I'm overextending in relationships. I'm practicing.

The sheer pain of this experience has also lit quite a fire under me. I have become extremely attentive and meticulous about doing everything in my power to prevent the mere possibility of ever developing another bladder infection as long as I live!

As it turns out I am, in fact, pregnant. I unknowingly conceived a few days prior to the onset of the illness. I believe it was the healing qualities and warmth of the abdominal wraps, the compresses and the home remedies that miraculously supported a new life, even under such extreme conditions.

As my example shows, the three paths of care already presented can clearly be interwoven to aid in the healing process. When someone's condition is worsening rapidly from an infection or inflammation, antibiotics can be crucial in readily eliminating the bacteria. Just as crucial is supporting the environment that the bacteria are growing in--your body! Home therapies and natural medicines can help by gently guiding your body back to a state of balance. Finally, directing and redirecting your attention back to your need for warmth, proper nutrition, rest, and fluids is what seems to truly allow the other interventions to be most effective.

6

A Reference Guide to Common Illnesses

TEMPLATE

∞ **DESCRIPTION AND SYMPTOMS OF EACH CONDITION.** What are you dealing with?

∞ **RULING OUT EMERGENCY.** At the onset, what symptoms indicate the need for immediate medical attention?

∞ **COURSE OF ILLNESS.** You have decided that it is safe to stay home. What can you expect?

∞ **SIGNS OF HEALING.** These indicate you are on the right track.

∞ **WARNING SIGNS.** After several days, what symptoms indicate the need for further medical attention?

CHOOSING A PATH OF CARE

∞ **PATH ONE: SUPPORTING THE HEALING PROCESS** describes how to support the body's own innate healing powers.

∞ **PATH TWO: HOME THERAPIES** includes healing plant and mineral substances to further support the healing process.

∞ **PATH THREE: COMMONLY PRESCRIBED DRUGS** indicates which prescribed pharmaceuticals might be recommended and their role in the healing process.

BLADDER INFECTION

(Urinary Tract Infection, UTI, or Cystitis)

DESCRIPTION AND SYMPTOMS

Inflammation of the bladder.

Any or all of the following symptoms may be present: burning during urination, painful urination, sense of urgency of urination, frequent need to urinate, sensation of incomplete bladder emptying, blood in urine, lower abdominal pain or cramping, and cloudy urine.

RULING OUT EMERGENCY

Back pain and/or fever may indicate the onset of a kidney infection. See your healthcare provider immediately and begin supporting the healing process. (See Kidney Infection.)

COURSE OF ILLNESS

The course of illness for bladder infections is variable. If you have mild to moderate symptoms, healing can be expected within five to seven days when following the suggestions below. Other people may experience intense, rapidly progressing symptoms that lead to high fever and back pain within a day or two. Although bladder infections may fully resolve with care, further measures are often necessary.

For many people, especially women, bladder infections begin in the late teens and early twenties and can recur often. With increased frequency of infection comes more severe, rapidly progressing symptoms and possible antibiotic resistance. Therefore, from the very first bladder infection, it is important to take great care in strengthening the entire urinary system. This is achieved through supporting the healing process and home therapies. Practicing prevention, as described below, is the best place to focus energy if you suffer from this condition.

SIGNS OF HEALING

Decreased frequency and discomfort during urination and decreased bladder tenderness and pain can indicate healing. Also, the urine will become more clear.

WARNING SIGNS

See your doctor if the following symptoms develop.

Vaginal or penile discharge in association with the above mentioned symptoms is more likely to indicate an infection of the vagina, urethra, or cervix. The discharge may be yellow or green or fowl smelling.

Inability to urinate is important to watch for. An infection that is not healing may lead to so much inflammation of the urethra that it actually blocks urinary flow. If it becomes increasingly difficult or impossible to urinate while caring for a bladder infection, this may indicate such a blockage and signal the need to see a healthcare provider immediately. A bladder obstruction is an emergency condition. Catheterization and antibiotics may be advised.

NOTE: If you are pregnant or diabetic, consult your healthcare provider immediately.

CHOOSING A PATH OF CARE

PATH ONE: SUPPORTING THE HEALING PROCESS

Our body's innate healing powers have the ability to overcome most imbalances and common illnesses. Caring for the whole person through proper nutrition, fluids, warmth, rest, and care of the senses are the most critical ways to address any illness. The early use of these care-giving measures enhances the patient's opportunity to come out of the illness stronger, with more antibodies and white blood cells to reduce the likelihood of recurrence. Even if remedies, antibiotics, or other pharmaceuticals are taken, these principles of care are still the key to supporting a deeper healing and must be continued until well-being is reestablished. Healing requires us to have the courage to step back from the busyness of life and care for ourselves and our loved ones. Overcoming an illness in this way can then lead to new-found personal and spiritual strength and development. Before reading further, go to the beginning of Section Five and review "Path One: Supporting the Healing Process."

In the case of a bladder infection, increased fluids, warmth, and rest are of primary importance. Drink plenty of cranberry juice and hot tea (bearberry or uva-ursi, if possible). Warmth can be applied by using a hot-water bottle directly over the bladder. Keeping warm clothing on, especially over the lower belly, is critical.

PREVENTION

The best way for women to heal a bladder infection is to prevent it in the first place by:

a) Wiping from front to back after urinating and defecating.

b) Washing and urinating before sexual intercourse.

c) Washing and urinating after sexual intercourse (in that order).

d) Wearing cotton underwear.

Nutrition: Alternating acidic foods for three days with alkaline foods for three days can create an environment unfavorable to the proliferation of bacteria in the urine.

Acid Phase: During the three day acid phase, take 250 milligrams of vitamin C three times a day and drink cranberry juice.

Alkaline Phase: During the three-day alkaline phase avoid meats, soft drinks, and anything making the urine acidic. Uva-ursi or bearberry leaf tea and a pinch of baking soda three times a day can help turn the urine alkaline. Continue until symptoms have been gone for a week.

PATH TWO: HOME THERAPIES

See the following substances in Section Eight: A Reference Guide to Home Therapies.

Chamomile: A warm abdominal wrap can bring soothing warmth and healing to the entire pelvic region.

Echinacea: The recommended dosage can be taken to help boost the immune system, especially if there are cold and flu-like symptoms with fatigue and depletion.

The following remedy is not covered in Section Eight. It can be ordered or purchased at most health food stores.

Thuja 3x: Take the recommended dose of this homeopathic remedy to aid systemic healing. For dosage suggestions see Section Eight.

PATH THREE: COMMONLY PRESCRIBED DRUGS

If the symptoms become overwhelming or intolerable, or if more complicated infections are suspected, antibiotics and bladder anesthetics can often work quickly and effectively to eliminate the bacteria and decrease pain. They may also be indicated for people who have a history of recurrent infections or diabetes.

Bactrim, ciprofloxacin, norfloxacin, and ampicillin are commonly-prescribed antibiotics. In otherwise healthy women, a three-day course is typically recommended. Men may require at least seven days of antibiotics.

Pyridium is often used as a fast-acting bladder anesthetic.

BRONCHITIS

DESCRIPTION AND SYMPTOMS

Acute bronchitis is an inflammation of the upper airways, which follows a respiratory tract infection, such as a common cold.

Symptoms include cough (initially dry and unproductive, then productive), fever, fatigue, aching muscles, coughing up blood, burning sensation in chest, wheezing or noisy breathing.

RULING OUT EMERGENCY

Extreme difficulty breathing or rapid breathing may indicate pneumonia and require seeing a healthcare practitioner or doctor. (See Pneumonia.)

COURSE OF ILLNESS

Acute bronchitis, in patients who are non-smokers with no underlying lung disease, generally runs its course within 10 to 15 days. Repeated clinical trials have shown that antibiotics do not shorten the duration of symptoms despite their continued overuse.[17]

Fever is typical for the first three to five days. But the cough can persist for the duration of the illness.

A mild, less frequent cough can last an additional week or two.

SIGNS OF HEALING

Decreasing frequency and intensity of the cough. Decrease in sputum production (mucus produced in the large airways that is coughed up).

WARNING SIGNS

See your doctor if the following symptoms develop.

Persistent cough that is worsening and becoming more painful with bloody sputum may indicate pneumonia.

Shortness of breath may indicate pneumonia or the stimulation of an asthma-like reaction.

Persistent fever over 101 degrees F., that is present past the fifth or sixth day of the illness, may indicate a progression to pneumonia.

CHOOSING A PATH OF CARE

PATH ONE: SUPPORTING THE HEALING PROCESS

Our body's innate healing powers have the ability to overcome most imbalances and common illnesses. Caring for the whole person through proper nutrition, fluids, warmth, rest, and care of the senses are the most critical ways to address any illness. The early use of these care-giving measures enhances the patient's opportunity to come out of the illness stronger, with more antibodies and white blood cells to reduce the likelihood of recurrence. Even if remedies, antibiotics or other pharmaceuticals are taken, these principles of care are still the key to supporting a deeper healing and must be continued until well-being is reestablished. Healing requires us to have the courage to step back from the busyness of life and care for ourselves and our loved ones. Overcoming an illness in this way can then lead to new-found personal and spiritual strength and development. Before reading further, go to the beginning of Section Five and review "Path One: Supporting the Healing Process."

PATH TWO: HOME THERAPIES

As in caring for colds, using inhalations, rubs, steams, and remedies can effectively relieve symptoms of bronchitis without unwanted side effects. See the following healing substances in Section Eight: A Reference Guide to Home Therapies.

Chamomile: Use an inhalation for a soothing, healing effect on the chest and nasal passages.

Cinnabar: Use as an oral or systemic remedy if there is a sore throat and/or congested sinus area.

Echinacea: The recommended dosage can be taken to help boost the immune system, especially if there are cold and flu-like symptoms with fatigue and depletion.

Eucalyptus:

Essential oil can be used for steams and room vaporizers.

Rub or massage can be administered to the throat, chest and back.

Lemon:

Leg compresses are helpful if fever is present.

Chest compresses can bring localized healing in the lungs and chest area.

Throat compresses can bring relief and healing of sore throat.

PATH THREE: COMMONLY PRESCRIBED DRUGS

Antibiotics like Bactrim and erythromycin are commonly recommended for bronchitis. They do not shorten the duration of the illness in non-smokers and people without underlying lung disease, except when the illness has already been present for over two weeks.

In general, cough expectorants should be used as opposed to cough suppressants. (Be careful, as some cough expectorates may cause drowsiness.) In the setting of bronchitis, suppressing a cough can delay the clearing of unwanted mucus and may lead to pneumonia. If a cough is so severe as to interfere with sleep, taking a suppressant like Robitussin DM for a few nights is a reasonable compromise. Sleep is the best healer in these cases.

COLDS

DESCRIPTION AND SYMPTOMS

The common cold is an inflammation of the nasal passages and/or upper airways.

Symptoms include nasal stuffiness, sneezing, scratchy throat, cough, hoarseness, malaise, headache, fever.

RULING OUT EMERGENCY

Flu-like symptoms: The onset of a cold can occasionally mimic a flu. The acute onset of a fever higher than 102 degrees F. with severe headache and severe body aches in association with the above-mentioned symptoms often indicates a flu is in progress. Although influenza is not a true emergency condition, the very young and very old may experience severe consequences. Caring for a flu at its onset can prevent further complications. (See Flu.)

COURSE OF ILLNESS

The symptoms of a cold often last three to ten days.

SIGNS OF HEALING

The fever often goes down first, followed by decreased cough and frequency of sneezing. Hoarseness is one of the last symptoms to return to normal. A mild cough may last an extra few days as well.

WARNING SIGNS

See your doctor if the following symptoms develop.

Yellow or green mucus with severe nasal congestion or facial pain:

A common myth about colds is that, if the mucus turns yellow or green, there must be a bacterial infection requiring antibiotics. Good research has shown that colored mucus is simply a reflection of the body's white blood cells dying in response to healing.[18] If the person is feeling better, colored mucus alone is not a warning sign. However, the presence of yellow or green mucus with increased facial or forehead pain and severe sinus congestion may indicate a sinus infection.

Shortness of breath: It is common for those with lung disorders to have a shortness of breath associated with coughs and cold. Be prepared to address these underlying conditions directly, which are not covered in this guide.

If there is no underlying lung disease, such as asthma, then shortness of breath may indicate the presence of pneumonia or bronchitis.

CHOOSING A PATH OF CARE

PATH ONE: SUPPORTING THE HEALING PROCESS

Our body's innate healing powers have the ability to overcome most imbalances and common illnesses. Caring for the whole person through proper nutrition, fluids, warmth, rest, and care of the senses are the most critical ways to address any illness. The early use of these care-giving measures enhances the opportunity to come out of the illness stronger, with more antibodies and white blood cells to reduce the likelihood of recurrence. Even if remedies, antibiotics or other pharmaceuticals are taken, these principles of care are still the key to supporting a deeper healing and must be continued until well-being is reestablished. Healing requires us to have the courage to step back from the busyness of life and care for ourselves and our loved ones. Overcoming an illness in this way can then lead to newfound personal and spiritual strength and development. Before reading further, go to the beginning of Section Five and review "Path One: Supporting the Healing Process."

PATH TWO: HOME THERAPIES

Inhalations, rubs, steams, and remedies can effectively relieve cold symptoms without unwanted side effects. See the following substances in Section Eight: A Reference Guide to Home Therapies.

Chamomile: Inhalations can bring a soothing healing effect to the chest and nasal passages.

Cinnabar: Can be taken as an oral or systemic remedy for a hot, red throat. Look first in the back of the throat for any white or pussy spots. If pus is present, see your doctor.

Echinacea: The recommended dosage can be taken to help boost the immune system, especially if there are cold and flu-like symptoms with fatigue and depletion.

Eucalyptus:

Essential oil can be added to steams and room vaporizers.

Rub or massage can be administered to the throat, chest, and back.

Lemon:

Leg compresses are helpful if fever is present.

Chest compresses can bring localized healing in the chest area.

Throat compresses can bring relief and healing of sore throat.

Lavender: Baths can help relieve restlessness and irritability.

PATH THREE: COMMONLY PRESCRIBED DRUGS

A common cold will heal spontaneously and resolve itself within three to ten days. Conventional, over-the-counter medicines are used to relieve the symptoms, but they do not shorten the duration of the symptoms or illness.

Zinc gluconate may be an exception, as the lozenges have been shown to shorten the duration of cold symptoms in adults.

Decongestants are most useful to relieve nasal congestion. But side effects may include insomnia, nervousness, heart palpitations, and increased blood pressure.

A runny nose and frequent sneezing can be helped by antihistamines. Antihistamines may bring on drowsiness, dry mouth, urinary retention, and blurred vision. Combined decongestants and antihistamines can also be purchased without a prescription.

Prescription antihistamines and decongestants add the benefit of either having longer duration of action or less sedating effects.

Antibiotics are typically overused in treating the common cold. They simply breed bacterial resistance, bring unwanted side effects, and increase the likelihood of reinfection.[19]

COUGH

DESCRIPTION AND SYMPTOMS

Coughs may accompany a myriad of conditions, not limited to but including colds, bronchitis, flu, pneumonia, lung cancer, asthma, chronic bronchitis, and acid reflux disease. They may be either dry or productive of clear to bloody sputum. They may come in fits or come continuously. Coughs may be deep or high pitched or barking as in cases of croup.

The scope of this book does not allow for an in-depth discussion on how to differentiate one type of cough from another. Let good common sense guide you. If a cough persists for over two weeks without improving significantly, you should certainly see a practitioner for further evaluation.

Whooping cough or pertussis: Whooping cough is a highly contagious bacterial disease, usually occurring in children younger than four years. The first stage is characterized by a gradual onset of sneezing, runny nose, and fatigue, in addition to a hacking nighttime cough. After about 10-14 days, the cough becomes more frequent and more intense, followed by the whoop (a hurried deep inspiration). This stage may be accompanied by thick secretions with vomiting and gagging and can last up to four weeks. Hospitalization may be recommended, especially for children under two years of age or adults over 65, since serious complications are more likely to occur in these cases.

Although whooping cough can be effectively cared for at home, it should be known that full recovery can take several weeks or even months and should be carefully monitored by a healthcare practitioner. It can be treated successfully with home therapies and may also require erythromycin-like oral antibiotics. As whopping cough is contagious, carriers should take appropriate precautions such as avoiding school, day care, work, and contact with babies for at least four weeks, or until symptoms have subsided.

RULING OUT EMERGENCY

Difficulty in breathing: No matter what the cause of the shortness of breath, it should be evaluated by a doctor. If the person has been diagnosed with lung disease and knows how to address it at home, that approach can safely be attempted as long as the expected response is achieved in a timely fashion.

COURSE OF ILLNESS

See specific illness (i.e., Cold, Bronchitis, Flu).

SIGNS OF HEALING

If it is a productive cough, it will become less productive and less frequent. A dry cough will become less frequent. If there has been a difficulty in coughing up phlegm, then the ability to do so can indicate healing.

WARNING SIGNS

Same as above, under Ruling Out Emergency.

CHOOSING A PATH OF CARE

PATH ONE: SUPPORTING THE HEALING PROCESS

Our body's innate healing powers have the ability to overcome most imbalances and common illnesses. Caring for the whole person through proper nutrition, fluids, warmth, rest, and care of the senses are the most critical ways to address any illness. The early use of these care-giving measures enhances the patient's opportunity to come out of the illness stronger, with more antibodies and white blood cells to reduce the likelihood of recurrence. Even if remedies, antibiotics, or other pharmaceuticals are taken, these principles of care are still the key to supporting a deeper healing and must be continued until well-being is reestablished. Healing requires us to have the courage to step back from the busyness of life and care for ourselves and our loved ones. Overcoming an illness in this way can then lead to new-found personal and spiritual strength and development. Before reading further, go to the beginning of Section Five and review "Path One: Supporting the Healing Process".

PATH TWO: HOME THERAPIES

See the following substances in Section Eight: A Reference Guide to Home Therapies.

Chamomile: An inhalation can bring a soothing healing effect to the chest and nasal passages.

Cinnabar: As an oral or systemic remedy, it can promote healing of a red, hot throat and congested sinus area.

Echinacea: The recommended dosage can be taken to help boost the immune system, especially if there are cold and flu-like symptoms with fatigue and depletion.

Eucalyptus:

Essential oil can be used in steams and room vaporizers.

Rub or massage can be administered to the throat, chest, and back.

Lemon:

Chest compresses can bring more localized healing in the chest area.

Throat compresses can help bring relief and healing of a sore throat.

Leg compresses can help if fever is present.

PATH THREE: COMMONLY PRESCRIBED DRUGS

Antibiotics like Bactrim and erythromycin are commonly recommended for coughs and bronchitis. They do not shorten the duration of the illness in non-smokers and people without underlying lung disease, except when the illness has already been present for over two weeks.

With colds and allergies, a decongestant and antihistamine can be used to halt post-nasal drip, which is a common cause of persistent cough.

DEHYDRATION

DESCRIPTION AND SYMPTOMS

Dehydration is a depletion of body fluids that occurs when fluids are lost from the gastrointestinal tract, urinary tract, and skin.

Symptoms include dry tongue and sunken eyes, dizziness or light-headedness when standing, rapid heart rate, disorientation.

RULING OUT EMERGENCY

If the following symptoms occur, in addition to those mentioned above, seek immediate medical attention.

Light-headedness and altered mental status may mean that the blood pressure has dropped too low to sustain healthy neurological functioning.

COURSE OF ILLNESS

Dehydration can be reversed at any time during the course of an illness by sufficient fluid intake. This can be accomplished orally, rectally, or intravenously.

SIGNS OF HEALING

Willingness to drink, return of appetite, increased vitality and color, and mental clarity all indicate healing.

WARNING SIGNS

See your doctor if the following symptoms develop.

Unwillingness to drink or vomiting may indicate dehydration. Once dehydration has set in, it can become increasingly difficult to drink and keep fluids down. Dehydration can actually stimulate nausea and vomiting. In this case, fluid may be administered rectally by enema at home (see Chamomile below). If the enema is not retained, then intravenous fluids at a hospital or clinic may be indicated

Temperature/Heart Rate Guide: A good rule of thumb for estimating the appropriate heart rate response to fever is to remember the heart rate should be 100 beats per minute for a temperature of 100 degrees F. Then add 10 beats per minute for every degree above 100 degrees F. For example, with a temperature of 103 degrees F., the heart rate should be 130 beats per minute. This formula only holds for adults, who generally have lower rates than children. If the heart rate is higher than expected, dehydration may be the cause.

CHOOSING A PATH OF CARE

PATH ONE: SUPPORTING THE HEALING PROCESS

Our body's innate healing powers have the ability to overcome most imbalances and common illnesses. Caring for the whole person through proper nutrition, fluids, warmth, rest, and care of the senses are the most critical ways to address any illness. The early use of these care-giving measures enhances the patient's opportunity to come out of the illness stronger, with more antibodies and white blood cells to reduce the likelihood of recurrence. Even if remedies, antibiotics, or other pharmaceuticals are taken, these principles of care are still the key to supporting a deeper healing and must be continued until well-being is reestablished. Healing requires us to have the courage to step back from the busyness of life and care for ourselves and our loved ones. Overcoming an illness in this way can then lead to new-found personal and spiritual strength and development. Before reading further, go to the beginning of Section Five and review "Path One: Supporting the Healing Process".

The best way to prevent dehydration is by drinking plenty of fluids immediately at the onset and throughout any illness, especially when fever, vomiting, and diarrhea are present. (If you are breastfeeding, encourage the child to nurse as often as possible.) See "Fluids" in Section Four.

PATH TWO: HOME THERAPIES

See the following substances in Section Eight: A Reference Guide to Home Therapies:

Chamomile: An enema can provide essential electrolytes and may promote calming and soothing of the lower intestine.

Fluids: See Section Four.

PATH THREE: COMMONLY PRESCRIBED DRUGS

Many over-the-counter antidiarrheals, such as Imodium and Lomotil, can help stop diarrhea. Compazine, Phenergan, and Tigan are antiemetics, which are often prescribed to decrease severe nausea and vomiting. Know that they can be taken orally, rectally, and through injection. This class of medicines can cause drowsiness and uncontrolled movement in five to ten% of cases.

DIARRHEA

DESCRIPTION AND SYMPTOMS

Abrupt onset of diarrhea is usually caused by an inflammatory process or ingestion of toxins. A variety of symptoms are often observed, including frequent passage of watery stool, fever, chills, vomiting, and malaise.

Symptoms include loose liquid stools, abdominal pain and distention, headache, loss of appetite, fatigue, muscle aches, cramping, and loss of weight.

RULING OUT EMERGENCY

Belly tenderness, in addition to the diarrhea, should be evaluated by a healthcare provider.

Bloody diarrhea requires immediate evaluation.

High fever over 103 degrees F., especially in the very young or elderly, requires evaluation.

COURSE OF ILLNESS

Most acute cases of diarrhea will resolve on their own after 24 to 72 hours.

SIGNS OF HEALING

Watch for firmer stools and resolution of above-mentioned symptoms.

WARNING SIGNS

See your doctor if the following symptoms develop.

Dry lips, dry mouth, nausea, and sunken eyes may indicate dehydration. Please seek a professional opinion. This is especially important in cases of severe diarrhea in the very young child or the older adult. (See Dehydration.)

CHOOSING A PATH OF CARE

PATH ONE: SUPPORTING THE HEALING PROCESS

Our body's innate healing powers have the ability to overcome most imbalances and common illnesses. Caring for the whole person through proper nutrition, fluids, warmth, rest, and care of the senses are the most critical ways to address any illness. The early use of these care-giving measures enhances the patient's opportunity to come out of the illness stronger, with more antibodies and white blood cells to reduce the likelihood of recurrence. Even if remedies, antibiotics, or other pharmaceuticals are taken, these principles of care are still the key to supporting a deeper healing and must be continued until well-being is reestablished. Healing requires us to have the courage to step back from the busyness of life and care for ourselves and our loved ones. Overcoming an illness in this way can then lead to new-found personal and spiritual strength and development. Before reading further, go to the beginning of Section Five and review "Path One: Supporting the Healing Process".

Nutrition and Fluid: Dr. Philip Incao's patient handout states:

"The most important measure for care of diarrhea is proper abstinence from food intake. In such conditions, the stomach and intestines are very inflamed and they will be irritated by any food which enters them, thus resulting in more diarrhea and cramps. However, the person must drink enough fluids to prevent dehydration, especially infants. In general breast feeding is always best. However, if a child is having difficulty keeping breast milk down, it may be best to stop breastfeeding for a short time and give only clear fluids.

When feeling much better, cream of rice cereal and clear vegetable broth can be eaten. If this is well tolerated, move toward an apple, rice, and soft, cooked vegetables like squash or carrots. Try to avoid eggs or dairy until there has been a complete recovery. If at any time the conditions worsen, then go back to the beginning and start again.

The general rule is that inflamed bowels will heal as long as they can have a rest from having to cope with food, or even too much to drink. If the diarrhea is not improving, then try eating less for a few hours and see if there is improvement."[20] (Also see "Fluids" in Section Four.)

PATH TWO: HOME THERAPIES

See the following substances in Section Eight: A Reference Guide to Home Therapies.

Chamomile:

Tea: Start with only one teaspoon repeated every twenty minutes. If symptoms persist, then drink nothing for a couple of hours. Allow sleep and try again later. As symptoms begin to improve, the chamomile tea or Pedialyte intake may be very carefully increased. (Pedialyte can be purchased at most drug stores.)

Abdominal wraps: These may also provide comfort and healing.

Carbo Betulae 3x: This remedy helps bind or absorb toxins or other substances that may be responsible for the diarrhea. It can also bind gases and air that cause bloating and discomfort while it helps relax cramped intestinal muscles.

PATH THREE: COMMONLY PRESCRIBED DRUGS

Antidiarrheals are prescribed in cases where dehydration exists and diarrhea continues. They include Imodium and Lomotil. Antibiotics are advised in cases of traveler's diarrhea, and with fever and diarrhea lasting for more than five to seven days. They include Flagyl, Bactrim, and Cipro.

EARACHE

I. Inner ear infection or labyrinthitis

II. Middle ear infection or acute otitis media

(Note: Swimmer's ear is not covered in this guide.)

I. INNER EAR INFECTION

DESCRIPTION AND SYMPTOMS

Inner ear infection or labyrinthitis is an inflammation of the vestibular system of the inner ear.

Symptoms include vertigo (an illusion of motion), hearing loss, nausea, vomiting, ringing in ears, and malaise. It most commonly occurs in adults.

RULING OUT EMERGENCY

The following symptoms require emergency evaluation:

Head trauma.

Facial droop.

Weakness of an arm or a leg.

Loss of coordination.

COURSE OF ILLNESS

Inner ear infection is usually associated with a mild common cold. It can last seven to ten days, and the vertigo can be very uncomfortable. Changing positions often increases or worsens the vertigo. There is usually no inner ear pain associated with this condition.

SIGNS OF HEALING

Resolution of vertigo and ringing in ears with return of hearing.

WARNING SIGNS

See your doctor if the symptoms do not improve within five to seven days.

If the above-mentioned symptoms are accompanied by pain, fever, or discharge, see Middle Ear Infection.

CHOOSING A PATH OF CARE

PATH ONE: SUPPORTING THE HEALING PROCESS

(Note: This discussion assumes the care of a physician.)

Our body's innate healing powers have the ability to overcome most imbalances and common illnesses. Caring for the whole person through proper nutrition, fluids, warmth, rest, and care of the senses are the most critical ways to address any illness. The early use of these care-giving measures enhances the patient's opportunity to come out of the illness stronger, with more antibodies and white blood cells to reduce the likelihood of recurrence. Even if remedies, antibiotics, or other pharmaceuticals are taken, these principles of care are still the key to supporting a deeper healing and must be continued until well-being is reestablished. Healing requires having the courage to step back from the busyness of life and care for ourselves and our loved ones. Overcoming an illness in this way can then lead to new-found personal and spiritual strength and development. Before reading further, go to the beginning of Section Five and review "Path One: Supporting the Healing Process".

Movement: It is important to move and change positions slowly.

Nutrition: Eating a low-salt diet (less than four grams of salt per day) may help decrease the fluid retention in the inner ear, thereby minimizing the vertigo.

PATH TWO: HOME THERAPIES

If there are cold symptoms present, see Colds.

PATH THREE: COMMONLY PRESCRIBED DRUGS

The only drugs that are prescribed for inner ear infection, such as meclizine, are aimed at minimizing the degree of vertigo. They are only indicated if relief from vertigo is desired. They do not shorten the duration of this condition. Side effects of these drugs include dry mouth, blurred vision, and sedation.

II. MIDDLE EAR INFECTION

DESCRIPTION AND SYMPTOMS

Middle ear infection or acute otitis media can be related to a bacterial infection or a viral upper respiratory infection or a cold.

Symptoms include earache, fever, nasal discharge, cough, decreased hearing, bleeding or discharge from the ear, and irritability. Peak incidence is between 6 to 12 months of age, especially in children who have not been breastfed or are in day care. Incidence declines after 7 years of age. Otitis media is less common in adults, but occurrences can be quite uncomfortable.

RULING OUT EMERGENCY

An emergency exists if the above-mentioned symptoms are present with:

Vertigo: If severe vertigo (an illusion of motion) is present, seeking further care is advised. There may be an extension of the infection from the middle ear to the inner ear. Antibiotics may be indicated.

Trauma: If there has been penetrating trauma to the ear drum (e.g., overzealous use of a Q-tip or other sharp object), then expert care is advised. Ear drums (tympanic membranes) ruptured from infection may heal on their own, but large ruptures may need surgical interventions to restore hearing. To be safe, seek professional advice.

COURSE OF ILLNESS

The natural course of this condition is that it will resolve itself on its own within 7-10 days, without any intervention. Discharge can also last this long.

As pain is the most common and prominent symptom, it is good to know that the pain usually resolves within 24 hours in 60 to 80% of the cases.

Mild hearing loss is generally the last symptom to resolve. This is due to the fluid buildup in the ear being reabsorbed slowly.

Nearly 30% of children with recurrent otitis media will have associated mild to moderate hearing loss as a result of persistent fluid in the middle ear. Sometimes even temporary hearing loss in young children can lead to learning difficulties. When fluid persists for more than six months with some hearing loss, many doctors suggest Tympanostomy tubes. Tubes can help restore hearing and improve learning deficiencies. Ear tubes can also clog, cause inflammation, and scar eardrums leading to permanent hearing loss. They should be reserved for situations where alternatives have been tried for 3 to 6 months without success.

Permanent hearing loss from acute otitis media is an extremely rare and unpredictable complication. In a large study of 4,860 children who did not receive antibiotics, there were no cases of permanent hearing loss. [22]

In about 20 % of untreated ear infections, the inflammation can build up and the ear drum may rupture to discharge the pus. After the pus has burst through, the pain disappears quickly. Luckily, the ear drum is designed to expand and contract. So, as a rule, ruptured ear drums usually heal up well. In the rare cases that do not, but persist in manifesting a chronic discharge from the ear, the cause is nearly always an inherent weakness of the membrane. [21]

SIGNS OF HEALING

Resolution of pain is the first sign of healing. This is followed by decreased fever, decreased pressure in the ear, and finally improved hearing. It is not uncommon for complete resolution of hearing loss to take up to two to three weeks.

WARNING SIGNS

Further intervention and antibiotics may be indicated if there is:

Pain: If pain within the ear continues for more than two to three days, or if pain develops behind the ear with swelling and tenderness, seek expert advice.

Fever: If a temperature of over 102 degrees F. persists for more than three days, see a physician.

Headache and neck stiffness: If these symptoms arise at any time during the illness, it is important to rule out meningitis.

Recurring infections: More than 2 or 3 episodes of middle ear infection within a six-month period may require an evaluation to assess the underlying cause.

Drainage: Green, yellow or brown fluid draining from the ear requires further evaluation.

CHOOSING A PATH OF CARE

PATH ONE: SUPPORTING THE HEALING PROCESS

Our body's innate healing powers have the ability to overcome most imbalances and common illnesses. Caring for the whole person through proper nutrition, fluids, warmth, rest, and care of the senses are the most critical ways to address any illness. The early use of these care-giving measures enhances the patient's opportunity to come out of the illness stronger, with more antibodies and white blood cells to reduce the likelihood of recurrence. Even if remedies, antibiotics, or other pharmaceuticals are taken, these principles of care are still the key to supporting a deeper healing and must be continued until well-being is reestablished. Healing requires us to have the courage to step back from the busyness of life and care for ourselves and our loved ones. Overcoming an illness in this way can then lead to new-found personal and spiritual strength and development. Before reading further, go to the beginning of Section Five and review "Path One: Supporting the Healing Process".

PATH TWO: HOME THERAPIES

See the following substances in Section Eight: A Reference Guide to Home Therapies.

Echinacea can be used to help strengthen the immune system, especially if cold and flu symptoms are present.

Levisticum aids in the healing of the middle ear by its ability to bring warmth and air into an inflamed, fluid-filled space. (Available by prescription only.)

Onion compresses help to loosen the painful congestion in the ear (just as an onion draws tears from the eye). It is also effective in promoting drainage of fluid behind the ear drum that can remain after an earache is gone.

PATH THREE: COMMONLY PRESCRIBED DRUGS

Ear infections are the number one cause of antibiotic use (and probably overuse) in children in America. Amoxicillin, Bactrim, and Ceclor are most commonly prescribed. Their only benefit may be their ability to decrease the amount of pain present, if it persists for three to five days in uncomplicated cases. They are not effective in decreasing pain on the first day. They do not shorten the duration of an uncomplicated middle ear infection.[22]

A combination of supporting the healing process using home therapies, and avoiding antibiotics may prevent chronic recurring infections and the need for tubes in the ears.

Tylenol, Auralgan (anesthetic ear drops) and decongestants are also used.

FEVER

(Also see "The Value of Fever" in Section Four.)

DESCRIPTION AND SYMPTOMS

Fever is an increase in body temperature beyond the person's normal baseline temperature (commonly 98.6 degrees Fahrenheit or 37 degrees Celsius).

Symptoms: Tactile body heat, red cheeks, chills, shaking or rigors, delirium, confusion, and fatigue.

RULING OUT EMERGENCY

Fever itself is rarely an emergency. However, the following conditions associated with fever may require immediate medical attention:

Febrile convulsions are associated with a lack of consciousness; eyes rolling back; clenched fists; rigorous, whole-body, rigid shaking; drooling; and tongue biting. These generalized convulsions rarely last longer than five minutes and often stop by themselves without specific treatment. After the convulsion the person frequently goes to sleep and wakes up fine. Convulsions are thought to be caused by rapidly increasing or decreasing temperature. A high fever alone does not cause febrile convulsions, and medicines like Tylenol and Motrin do not prevent them.

If a seizure or convulsion does occur, put the person on his or her stomach, turn the head to one side, and make sure the mouth is empty. After the convulsion is complete, begin to bring down the temperature with leg compresses. (See Lemon in Section Eight.) A healthcare practitioner should be seen after any convulsion or seizure. See "Further Reading" to learn more about fever and convulsions.

Cold shock is a temperature rising above 104 degrees F. with altered mental status, while the skin remains cool.

Meningitis is associated with severe headache that persists after the temperature has risen, accompanied by retching or vomiting. (See Meningitis.)

COURSE OF ILLNESS

In general, there is usually an underlying cause behind a fever. It is often an inflammatory process such as a cold, flu, sinusitis, or inflammation of the skin, lung, or bladder. The source may also be due to an inflammatory process like rheumatoid arthritis, gout, or even cancer. Signs and symptoms of an underlying condition often manifest within a day or two after the onset of a fever. Knowing the source of a fever can bring peace of mind and help determine how to proceed most appropriately.

Assessing the Fever

In judging the progress of a fever, it is important to remember that behavior is more significant than the actual temperature. Watch the person closely to observe any change, or development of unusual behavior.

Another way of assessing the progress of a fever is to compare the body and limbs for warmth. If the limbs and calves feel cold, and the thermometer registers only 101.5 degrees F., the temperature is likely to continue to rise. Calves and feet will only become warm just before the temperature has stopped rising and the body is ready to disperse warmth. Therefore, do not apply leg compresses before that stage has been reached. Cover the person warmly and give plenty of warm or hot herb tea.

If the skin is hot right down to the calves and the temperature is over 102 degrees F., then leg compresses may be applied to help disperse surplus heat through the skin.[23] (See Lemon in Section Eight.)

SIGNS OF HEALING

Watch for decreased temperature and resolution of underlying condition.

WARNING SIGNS

If the temperature is decreasing without resolution of other symptoms, this may indicate the need for medical evaluation.

See Dehydration in this section.

CHOOSING A PATH OF CARE

PATH ONE: SUPPORTING THE HEALING PROCESS

Our body's innate healing powers have the ability to overcome most imbalances and common illnesses. Caring for the whole person through proper nutrition, fluids, warmth, rest, and care of the senses are the most critical ways to address any illness. The early use of these care-giving measures enhances the patient's opportunity to come out of the illness stronger, with more antibodies and white blood cells to reduce the likelihood of recurrence. Even if remedies, antibiotics, or other pharmaceuticals are taken, these principles of care are still the key to supporting a deeper healing and must be continued until well-being is reestablished. Healing requires us to have the courage to step back from the busyness of life and care for ourselves and our loved ones. Overcoming an illness in this way can then lead to new-found personal and spiritual strength and development. Before reading further, go to the beginning of Section Five and review "Path One: Supporting the Healing Process".

> **Nourishment** is very important during a fever. While the temperature is rising, the appetite is usually decreased. This is the time to give plenty of warm broths and hot teas. Once the fever is established, especially if there is no diarrhea, continue to give plenty of fluids and light

foods. Try to avoid too much fat and protein, as these are difficult to digest while the body is trying to heal.

PATH TWO: HOME THERAPIES

See the following substances in Section Eight: A Reference Guide to Home Therapies. Other remedies may be appropriate, depending on the underlying condition. See Cold, Flu, Bronchitis, etc.

TO DISSIPATE FEVER

Lemon leg compresses: If a child or adult with a high fever is uncomfortable and restless, then a lemon leg compress may be applied.

Arnica rub or massage: As a last resort, you may rub the arms, legs, and head with a washcloth moistened with tepid water and arnica essence. Rub vigorously to make the skin red, and this will help to dissipate excess body heat through the skin. If possible, keep the person warm from the neck to the knees during this process.

TO INCREASE FEVER

Hot baths: Sometimes the illness may be prolonged because the body is not producing enough fever to accomplish its purpose. Therefore, when an illness persists, and the fever stays rather low (99 or 100 F.), hot baths may be helpful.

In the evening, just before going to bed, sit in a hot bath for about 20 minutes. Keep adding more hot water to the bath until the temperature reaches 101 F., or until you can't tolerate the heat anymore. Wrap up warmly and jump into bed under lots of blankets. Then go to sleep without getting up again. This can be repeated every evening until the illness is "burned out."

CAUTION: It is important to have assistance with this bath, as you may feel faint or dizzy, especially when getting out. Get out very slowly and carefully. If you feel dizzy, sit down and put your head down between your legs. Very hot baths are only recommended for young, healthy people

PLACE
STAMP
HERE

Anthroposophic Press
3390 Route 9
Hudson, NY 12534-9420 USA

ℰ ANTHROPOSOPHIC PRESS

www.anthropress.org

PHONE: 518-851-2054

FAX: 800-925-1795

E-MAIL: service@anthropress.org

We publish and distribute the works of Rudolf Steiner, anthroposophy, and related authors. For more information and a current catalog, please check the appropriate boxes, fill in your name and address, and return this card.

SPECIAL INTERESTS:

☐ Agriculture (BD)
☐ Art/Literature (ART)
☐ Books for Children (CHILD)
☐ Crafts & Activities (FAM)
☐ Education (EDUC)
☐ Health (HEAL)
☐ Personal Development (INDEV)
☐ Science (SCIE)
☐ Social Transformation (SOC)
☐ Spiritual Science & Rudolf Steiner (ES)

NAME..

ADDRESS..

CITY/STATE..

ZIP/COUNTRY....................................

PHONE...

E-MAIL..

COMMENTS...

....

....

....

☐ Please do not make my name available to other organizations

I found this card in the book entitled *Healing at Home*

with strong hearts and should not be used during pregnancy.[24]

PATH THREE: COMMONLY PRESCRIBED DRUGS

Antipyretics like Tylenol and Motrin can help decrease the temperature and discomfort. Phenobarbital is often recommended for generalized seizures. A further discussion of prescribed drugs is beyond the scope of this book . See your healthcare practitioner.

FLU

(Influenza)

DESCRIPTION AND SYMPTOMS

Influenza is an acute illness typically associated with influenza A virus. It is marked by fever and inflammation of the nose, throat, eyes, and respiratory tract.

Symptoms include sudden onset of high fever, muscle aches that can last for days, sore throat, nonproductive cough, headache, swollen neck lymph nodes, chills, nasal congestion, runny nose, and sneezing.

RULING OUT EMERGENCY

Severe headache, rash, or stiff neck with change in mental status may indicate the need for immediate medical assistance. (See Meningitis.)

COURSE OF ILLNESS

Flu starts with a rapid onset of symptoms and tends to resolve on its own within 7 to 10 days. Body aches tend to resolve last.

SIGNS OF HEALING

Resolution of symptoms.

WARNING SIGNS

If the following symptoms develop while at home, then further medical attention is advised:

Non-productive cough with shortness of breath, may indicate the onset of influenza pneumonia.

Productive cough with shortness of breath, may indicate bacterial pneumonia that often complicates the course in older adults.

Severe headaches with stiff neck or altered mental status could indicate meningitis. Seek professional attention. (See Meningitis.)

CHOOSING A PATH OF CARE

PATH ONE: SUPPORTING THE HEALING PROCESS

Our body's innate healing powers have the ability to overcome most imbalances and common illnesses. Caring for the whole person through proper nutrition, fluids, warmth, rest, and care of the senses are the most critical ways to address any illness. The early use of these care-giving measures enhances the patient's opportunity to come out of the illness stronger, with more antibodies and white blood cells to reduce the likelihood of recurrence. Even if remedies, antibiotics, or other pharmaceuticals are taken, these principles of care are still the key to supporting a deeper healing and must be continued until well-being is reestablished. Healing requires us to have the courage to step back from the busyness of life and care for ourselves and our loved ones. Overcoming an illness in this way can then lead to new-found personal and spiritual strength and development. Before reading further, go to the beginning of Section Five and review "Path One: Supporting the Healing Process".

PATH TWO: HOME THERAPIES

For the flu, as for colds and coughs, inhalations, rubs, steams and remedies can effectively relieve symptoms without unwanted side effects. See the following substances in Section Eight: A Reference Guide to Home Therapies.

Chamomile: An inhalation can bring relief to a chest cough and stuffy nose.

Echinacea: The recommended dosage can be taken to help boost the immune system, especially if there are cold and flu-like symptoms with fatigue and depletion.

Eucalyptus:

Essential oil can be used in steams and room vaporizers.

Rub or massage can be administered to the throat, chest, and back.

Infludoron: This systemic remedy is taken orally to strengthen the immune response in the head region and associated mucus membranes.

Lemon:

Leg compresses can be helpful if fever is present.

Chest compresses can be used for more localized healing in the chest area.

Throat compresses can bring relief and healing of sore throat.

Lavender: A soothing bath can help relieve restlessness and irritability.

PATH THREE: COMMONLY PRESCRIBED DRUGS

The flu virus is one of the few viruses for which there is a specific antiviral agent that decreases the intensity and shortens the duration of symptoms. For instance, Amantadine, if given within the first 48 hours, can be helpful in achieving these goals. Unfortunately, it may bring on the following side effects: numbness, tingling and pain in the limbs, seizures, and altered mental status.

There is also a flu vaccine available. The virus changes from year to year; therefore, every fall a new vaccine is created. Some health organizations recommend the vaccine for people over 65; people who have chronic heart, lung, kidney, or liver disease; and healthcare professionals. These people may have an increased risk of pneumonia.

KIDNEY INFECTION

(Pyelonephritis)

DESCRIPTION AND SYMPTOMS

Pyelonephritis represents a deep-seated inflammation in one or both kidneys. Once these vital organs are infected, the accompanying inflammation is generally painful and hard to help resolve. Fever, painful urination (dysuria), mid- to low-back pain, increased frequency of urination, malaise, and nausea are typical. It can occur without any urinary symptoms as back pain, nausea or fever.

RULING OUT EMERGENCY

Fever over 103 degrees F. with altered mental status or light-headedness may indicate a blood infection that requires immediate administration of an antibiotic.

COURSE OF ILLNESS

There can be very slow healing over a two to three week period. Fever is expected for three to five days, and the back pain can take up to a week or two to fully resolve. It is best treated in the early stages.

In general, pyelonephritis requires the direct aid of a healthcare practitioner and antibiotic use. A kidney infection does not mean hospitalization is necessary, although some people do get hospitalized.

SIGNS OF HEALING

A gradual decline in temperature is expected along with temperature spikes nightly. These spikes should become lower and lower until the fever has fully disappeared.

WARNING SIGNS

Seek medical attention if the following symptoms develop:

Severe nausea and vomiting can prohibit oral intake, especially antibiotic intake.

Intractable back pain unresponsive to oral pain medications and topical applications should be evaluated.

Dehydration may be present if the mouth is dry, and the heart rate over 120 beats per minute with a temperature less than 102 degrees F.

CHOOSING A PATH OF CARE

PATH ONE: SUPPORTING THE HEALING PROCESS

(Note: This discussion assumes the care of a qualified healthcare practitioner.)

Our body's innate healing powers have the ability to overcome most imbalances and common illnesses. Caring for the whole person through proper nutrition, fluids, warmth, rest, and care of the senses are the most critical ways to address any illness. The early use of these care-giving measures enhances the patient's opportunity to come out of the illness stronger, with more antibodies and white blood cells to reduce the likelihood of recurrence. Even if remedies, antibiotics, or other pharmaceuticals are taken, these principles of care are still the key to supporting a deeper healing and must be continued until well-being is reestablished. Healing requires us to have the courage to step back from the busyness of life and care for ourselves and our loved ones. Overcoming an illness in this way can then lead to new-found personal and spiritual strength and development. Before reading further, go to the beginning of Section Five and review "Path One: Supporting the Healing Process".

Fluids: Enough cannot be said about the importance of fluid intake in healing this condition. Whether or not antibiotics are being used, fluids, rest, warmth, and local compresses and applications are truly needed for full recovery and healing without relapse.

Nutrition: Alternating acidic foods for three days with alkaline foods for three days can create an unfavorable living environment for bacteria in the urine.

Acid Phase: During the three-day acid phase, take 250 milligrams of vitamin C three times a day and drink cranberry juice.

Alkaline Phase: During the three-day alkaline phase, avoid meats, soft drinks and anything making the urine acidic. Uva ursi or bearberry leaf tea and a pinch of baking soda, in a glass of water, three times a day can help turn the urine alkaline. Continue until symptoms have been gone for a week.

PATH TWO: HOME THERAPIES

(Note: With a kidney infection, the following suggestions should always be supervised by a qualified healthcare practitioner.)

See the following substances in Section Eight: A Reference Guide to Home Therapies.

Chamomile: Abdominal compresses can bring soothing warmth and aid in the healing of the entire lower abdomen and bladder.

Echinacea: The recommended dosage can be taken to help boost the immune system, especially if there are cold and flu-like symptoms with fatigue and depletion.

Lavender: Baths can bring relief to restlessness and irritability.

Lemon: Leg compresses can be helpful if fever is present.

For more severe cases, where extra healing support is needed, the following substances can be helpful. Although they are not covered in Section Eight, they can be ordered through the companies listed in the "Resources" section at the end of the book.

Cuprum: Ointment brings a harmonizing effect when applied to the skin overlying the kidneys. It also brings warmth to support healing.

Equisetum: Compresses do much the same thing but also provide the kidney with restorative forces that bring added structure to the almost literally dissolving, inflamed kidneys. Ingesting equisetum tea internalizes these healing properties. This combination of methods allows the kidneys to be strengthened from inside and out.

PATH THREE: COMMONLY PRESCRIBED DRUGS

As with most infections, antibiotics are the only drugs uniformly prescribed. Cipro, Norflox, and Bactrim are the ones most commonly used. Antibiotics are usually required for up to two weeks, because of the deep-seated nature of the infection.

MASTITIS

DESCRIPTION AND SYMPTOMS

Mastitis is an inflammation of the breast duct or ducts. It may be preceded by a clogged duct.

Symptoms include sore or tender lump in one or both breasts, a red area on the skin, painful nursing, fatigue, sudden high fever (over 101 degrees F.), and chills.

RULING OUT EMERGENCY

See "Warning Signs" below.

COURSE OF ILLNESS

Because the breast tissue is such a highly vascular system, infection can spread very rapidly. Fever can spike very quickly after the onset of symptoms. So, despite the method of care, symptoms can seem worse before they get better. Improvement can normally be expected within the first 24 to 36 hours.

SIGNS OF HEALING

Watch for decreasing fever. Lump and tenderness should subside.

WARNING SIGNS

If the following additional symptoms develop after the first two or three days, medical attention is advised. These symptoms may indicate that an abscess has formed. These conditions are very serious and may require surgical drainage or removal of the lump.

Enlarged lump that is not going down or that is spreading with more redness under armpit or toward breastbone.

Unrelenting fever that continues to spike over 102 degrees F.

CHOOSING A PATH OF CARE

PATH ONE: SUPPORTING THE HEALING PROCESS

Our body's innate healing powers have the ability to overcome most imbalances and common illnesses. Caring for the whole person through proper nutrition, fluids, warmth, rest, and care of the senses are the most critical ways to address any illness. The early use of these care-giving measures enhances the patient's opportunity to come out of the illness stronger, with more antibodies and white blood cells to reduce the likelihood of recurrence. Even if remedies, antibiotics, or other pharmaceuticals are taken, these principles of care are still the key to supporting a deeper healing and must be continued until well-being is reestablished. Healing requires us to have the courage to step back from the busyness of life and care for ourselves and our loved ones. Overcoming an illness in this way can then lead to new-found personal and spiritual strength and development. Before reading further, go to the beginning of Section Five and review "Path One: Supporting the Healing Process".

Since mastitis can spread very quickly, it is important to begin care immediately after the first sign of infection.

Sleep or at least rest with the baby as often as possible!

Drink as much as possible.

Stay warm with a hot-water bottle by your feet or abdomen.

Nurse as often as possible, even though there may be nipple tenderness.

Bathe between naps, submersing and soaking the breasts.

Massage the sore breast before nursing with clean hands. Use a very gentle circular motion going from the outside of the breast toward the nipple. Begin the massage at the furthest point away from the lump or tender area. End with a very light and gentle motion over the lump itself.

Wear loose cotton clothing with no bra.

PATH TWO: HOME THERAPIES

See the following substances in Section Eight: A Reference Guide to Home Therapies.

Cottage cheese compresses can help draw the infection to the surface and move it out of the breast.

Echinacea can be taken in remedy form to help boost the immune system, especially if there are cold and flu symptoms present.

Lemon leg compresses can help with the discomfort of a high fever.

PATH THREE: COMMONLY PRESCRIBED DRUGS

Antibiotics are most commonly prescribed for a breast infection and may be indicated if the symptoms are getting worse after two or three days. Two of the antibiotics used for mastitis, Keflex and dicloxacillin, are also used for treating streptoccocal and staphylococcal infections.

MENINGITIS

DESCRIPTION AND SYMPTOMS

Meningitis is an inflammation of the membranes covering the brain and spinal cord.

There are two kinds of meningitis: bacterial and viral.

a) Bacterial meningitis is an inflammation of the lining of the brain and spinal cord, which is caused by a bacterial infection. It is considered a medical emergency. It is rare.

b) Viral meningitis is a viral infection of the membrane layers covering the brain and spinal cord.

Symptoms include a marked change in behavior during the course of a fever, stiff neck, severe headache, inflammation of deep lymph nodes in the neck, sensitivity to light, rash, nausea, and vomiting.

RULING OUT EMERGENCY

If any of the above-mentioned symptoms occurs during the course of a fever, immediate medical attention is critical.

To test for meningitis, have the ill person:

a) Sit up in bed with the legs straight out and raise the outstretched arms. If there is difficulty in sitting up properly, leaning back on the arms with the head tilted back, or if there is difficulty bringing the arms forward without pain in the head and back, then meningitis is probably present.

b) Sit up, bend the knee, and try to touch it with the mouth. If this is difficult and produces pain in the head and back, it indicates the possibility of meningitis. [23]

HEALING AT HOME

(Note: This discussion assumes the care of a qualified healthcare practitioner.)

Meningitis is a rare but serious, life-threatening illness that usually requires hospitalization and sometimes intensive care. Trust your instincts! If you detect even the slightest indication of its presence, immediately have the ill person diagnosed by a qualified healthcare practitioner. To further help a person with meningitis, see: "Path One: Supporting the Healing Process" in Section Five and "Flu " in Section Six.

PNEUMONIA

DESCRIPTION AND SYMPTOMS

Pneumonia is an inflammation of the lung.

Symptoms include cough and fever; chest pain; chills with sudden onset; productive cough, spitting up thick or bloody mucus or sputum; abnormal heart rate; rapid breathing; bluish discoloration around eyes, lips, and nails; changes in levels of consciousness; anxiety; confusion; and restlessness; abdominal pain and loss of appetite; profuse sweating; muscle aches; and dark red lips.

RULING OUT EMERGENCY

If the following symptoms are present at the onset of the illness, then immediate medical attention is advised:

Shortness of breath, bluish coloring around the lips, altered mental status may indicate a lack of oxygen in the blood.

Severe chest pain on inhalation requires an evaluation.

COURSE OF ILLNESS

Healing generally takes 10 to 14 days, although the abnormal signs seen on x ray may not fully resolve for up to 6 weeks.

Pneumonia can be dangerous in the elderly, in infants and in delicate children and adults. Otherwise, it is not necessarily a life-threatening illness. Treatment should be supervised by a healthcare practitioner, and hospitalization may be required.

CHOOSING A PATH OF CARE

PATH ONE: SUPPORTING THE HEALING PROCESS

(Note: This discussion assumes the care of a healthcare practitioner.)

Our body's innate healing powers have the ability to overcome most imbalances and common illnesses. Caring for the whole person through proper nutrition, fluids, warmth, rest, and care of the senses are the most critical ways to address any illness. The early use of these care-giving measures enhances the patient's opportunity to come out of the illness stronger, with more antibodies and white blood cells to reduce the likelihood of recurrence. Even if remedies, antibiotics, or other pharmaceuticals are taken, these principles of care are still the key to supporting a deeper healing and must be continued until well-being is reestablished. Healing requires us to have the courage to step back from the busyness of life and care for ourselves and our loved ones. Overcoming an illness in this way can then lead to new-found personal and spiritual strength and development. Before reading further, go to the beginning of Section Five and review "Path One: Supporting the Healing Process".

PATH TWO: HOME THERAPIES

See the following substances in Section Eight: A Reference Guide to Home Therapies. The goal with home therapies is to help expectorate or cough up the pus in the lungs. Doing so will help eliminate the shortness of breath.

Chamomile: Inhalations and humidity can help with healing. The air quality in the room should be as fresh and light as possible without causing a draft.

Cottage cheese: If there is considerable accumulation of fluid in the lungs, use a warm, damp compress with curd cheese on the chest.

Echinacea: In remedy form this can help strengthen the immune system.

Eucalyptus:

Essential oil can be used in steams and room vaporizers.

Rub or massage can be administered to the throat, chest and back.

Lavender baths can help soothe restlessness and irritability.

Lemon:

Leg compresses can be helpful if fever is present.

Chest compresses promote localized healing in the chest area.

Throat compress can bring relief and healing of sore throat.

PATH THREE: COMMONLY PRESCRIBED DRUGS

Antibiotics are the mainstay for this condition. Ceftin, Augmentin, Zithromax and Biaxin are most commonly used when hospitalization is not required. Expectorants and cough suppressants like Robitussin and Dextromethorphan are also used.

A vaccine is available for people over 65; people with heart, lung liver, or kidney disease; and people who have had a spleenectomy.

SORE THROAT

(Pharyngitis)

DESCRIPTION AND SYMPTOMS

Sore throat, or pharyngitis, is an inflammation most commonly associated with the presence of a bacteria or virus.

Symptoms include enlarged tonsils; enlarged lymph nodes in the neck; absence of cough, hoarseness, or lower respiratory symptoms; fever over 102.5 degrees F., rash, loss of appetite, chills, headache, and reddened eyes.

RULING OUT EMERGENCY

If the following symptoms are present at the onset of a sore throat, then seek immediate medical care.

Obstructed throat and airways making it very difficult to breath, eat, or drink. This may indicate an enlarged epiglottis (the flap of tissue in the lower throat that protects the airway when swallowing).

COURSE OF ILLNESS

The course of pharyngitis varies, depending on the source of inflammation. A sore throat is most often due to a viral infection with the onset of soreness occurring over a gradual period of one to two days. It can be accompanied by a slight fever, cough, runny nose, and hoarseness.

Sore throat is less often associated with a swiftly emerging bacterial infection (like strep), accompanied by redness, pus, and generally an absence of cough.

Strep throat can be detected by looking for the following three symptoms: pus on the tonsils and in the back and sides of the throat, swollen glands in the neck, and a temperature of above 101 degrees F. Pus is present when a normally pink throat appears to be fiery red, with spots of white or yellow that often look like cottage cheese.

These symptoms can persist for three to five days without requiring further medical attention.

SIGNS OF HEALING

Watch for relief of symptoms.

WARNING SIGNS

If the sore throat persists for more than five days, then further medical care is advised. A throat culture and blood test may be indicated to rule out mononucleosis, leukemia, diphtheria, or other conditions.

CHOOSING A PATH OF CARE

PATH ONE: SUPPORTING THE HEALING PROCESS

Our body's innate healing powers have the ability to overcome most imbalances and common illnesses. Caring for the whole person through proper nutrition, fluids, warmth, rest, and care of the senses are the most critical ways to address any illness. The early use of these care-giving measures enhances the patient's opportunity to come out of the illness stronger, with more antibodies and white blood cells to prevent likelihood of recurrence. Even if remedies, antibiotics, or other pharmaceuticals are taken, these principles of care are still the key to supporting a deeper healing and must be continued until well-being is reestablished. Healing requires us to have the courage to step back from the busyness of life and care for ourselves and our loved ones. Overcoming an illness in this way can then lead to new-found personal and spiritual strength and development. Before reading further, go to the beginning of Section Five and review "Path One: Supporting the Healing Process".

PATH TWO: HOME THERAPIES

See the following substances in Section Eight: A Reference Guide to Home Therapies.

Cinnabar: This remedy can help in the healing process of the red, hot throat. (It is not to be used if there is pus in the throat.)

Echinacea:

Remedy form can help strengthen the immune system.

Eucalyptus:

Essential oil can be used in steams and room vaporizers.

Rub or massage can be administered to the throat, chest and back.

Lavender: Baths can help relieve restlessness and irritability.

Lemon:

Leg compresses can help if fever is present.

Chest compresses promote localized healing in the chest area.

Throat compresses can bring relief and healing of sore throat.

PATH THREE: COMMONLY PRESCRIBED DRUGS

Antibiotics may be indicated for certain bacterial infections. Viscous lidocaine may be prescribed to anesthetize the back of the throat to ease swallowing and prevent dehydration.

STOMACHACHE

DESCRIPTION AND SYMPTOMS

Abdominal pain caused by indigestion, food allergies, or medications; or experienced as the by-product of another ailment.

RULING OUT EMERGENCY

If there is abdominal pain (with tenderness to the touch) accompanied by the following symptoms, further medical advice is advised:

Vomiting blood, diarrhea, bloody stools, persistent loss of appetite, weight loss, severe abdominal pain and fever.

Appendicitis is usually accompanied by vomiting and fever, but the vomiting may not be persistent, and the fever may be very mild. In the early stages of appendicitis, the pain is usually generalized throughout the entire abdomen. Within a matter of hours it will localize in the lower-right quadrant. Pressure at that point will cause intense pain. If the appendix ruptures, the pain will again become generalized throughout the abdomen. An appendicitis attack is almost always preceded by a lack of appetite. Blood tests and surgery may be indicated.

SIGNS OF HEALING

Look for resolution of symptoms and abdominal pain.

WARNING SIGNS

Severe abdominal pain that recurs repeatedly, or persists for more than two or three days, deserves further medical attention. The recommendations below are appropriate for occasional acute occurrences.

CHOOSING A PATH OF CARE

PATH ONE: SUPPORTING THE HEALING PROCESS

Our body's innate healing powers have the ability to overcome most imbalances and common illnesses. Caring for the whole person through proper nutrition, fluids, warmth, rest, and care of the senses are the most critical ways to address any illness. The early use of these care-giving measures enhances the patient's opportunity to come out of the illness stronger, with more antibodies and white blood cells to reduce the likelihood of recurrence. Even if remedies, antibiotics, or other pharmaceuticals are taken, these principles of care are still the key to supporting a deeper healing and must be continued until well-being is reestablished. Healing requires us to have the courage to step back from the busyness of life and care for ourselves and our loved ones. Overcoming an illness in this way can then lead to new-found personal and spiritual strength and development. Before reading further, go to the beginning of Section Five and review "Path One: Supporting the Healing Process".

PATH TWO: HOME THERAPIES

See the following substances in Section Eight: A Reference Guide to Home Therapies.

Carbo betulae can help absorb toxins in the abdomen and relieve symptoms.

Chamomile abdominal compress can bring soothing warmth and healing to discomfort and cramping in the abdomen.

Peppermint tea can help with indigestion. It can be purchased at most grocery stores.

PATH THREE: COMMONLY PRESCRIBED DRUGS

These will depend upon the underlying disorder and are too varied to adequately discuss here.

VACCINATIONS

Yes. No...........Maybe!

We are all led to believe that vaccinations are a mandatory, miraculous, safe and guaranteed method of avoiding very scary, life-threatening illnesses. As we investigated more, we discovered:

a) There is a choice.

b) There are serious side effects and risks associated with vaccinations.

c) They do not guarantee immunity.

d) Vaccinations introduce foreign proteins into the body and one cannot know the long-term consequences on the immune system.

The best way to make a decision is to read, read, read (see Further Reading in the appendix). If possible, become informed before you have children and are caught off guard at your first visit with your baby's pediatrician. It's an issue that has compelling arguments and intense feelings on both sides, so it's normal to feel confused or unsure. Postpone making a final decision until you can apply what you know to the specific child, and the specific environment and situation. Let that be your guide. Here are some arguments for and against having your children vaccinated.

YES:

Some of the considerations in deciding to vaccinate include your answers to questions such as these: Do you feel knowledgable about and comfortable with caring for a child experiencing a childhood illness? Can you take the time to do so? Do you live on a farm or in an area with a greater risk of exposure to tetanus? Will you soon travel to another country? What is the law in your state?

If you do choose to fully vaccinate, there are several things you can do to minimize unwanted side effects.

a) Wait until a child is well with no underlying cold or sore throat before vaccinating.

b) Consider arranging for the vaccines to be given separately instead of all at once. It means more pricks, but it may be less likely to overwhelm the system and cause unwanted systemic side effects. Individual vaccinations are available, but you may have to persevere to get them.

c) After a vaccination, care for a child by supporting the healing process, as if he or she had just been exposed to a virus or foreign protein. This will help the immune system cope with the vaccination and prevent unwanted side effects. See "Supporting the Healing Process" in Section Five.

d) Home therapies can also help the system cope with and potentially prevent unwanted side effects (see Section Eight).

Thuja, taken orally three times a day for a few days after the vaccination, can help prevent unwanted side effects. (This remedy is available at most health food stores in liquid and pellets. See dosage suggestions in Section Eight.)

Arnica compresses, applied locally to the site of the injection, can help with localized reactions.

NO:

Beyond the known physical risks of vaccinations, many people choose not to vaccinate for social, political, or religious reasons. For instance, the chicken pox vaccine was partially developed so working parents could stay at work and not have to take leave to care for a sick child. Some feel that if a child goes through an illness such as chicken pox, his or her immune system and developmental forces are strengthened.

If you choose not to immunize your children, then it is important to be very well versed in childhood illnesses. It is even more important to be prepared for and comfortable with the practical aspects of caring for a child while they are suffering from an illness. Whooping cough, for instance, can last several weeks and can take a lot of energy to care for.

The most important thing to be aware of is your level of fear of contracting one of these viruses. Do you have a support system of friends, relatives and professionals that can support you if you should contract such an illness? Could you bring a calm, healing presence to the situation? It is possible, believe it or not. It's just very difficult with the fear of disease that pervades our culture. Where do you stand?

MAYBE:

Who are the children? Are they predisposed to seizures or encephalitis? How healthy are their immune systems? What is the likelihood of their contracting each particular illness in your geographical area? Are they at high risk of being exposed to the virus? Do you have a positive relationship with a healthcare provider who could support the family through an illness? Which illnesses would be most difficult for you to manage at home? Is it possible to get some vaccinations and not others? Could some of the vaccinations, like hepatitis B, wait until the children are older?

Revisit these questions with each child and with each relocation or major shift in your family circumstance.

See the "Resources" and "Further Reading" sections in the appendix.

7

BASIC FIRST AID

```
┌──────────────────────────────────────────┐
│                                          │
│              TEMPLATE                     │
│              ─────────                    │
│                                          │
│   ∞ DESCRIPTION OF CONDITION              │
│                                          │
│   ∞ ACTION                                │
│                                          │
│   ∞ HOME REMEDIES                         │
│                                          │
└──────────────────────────────────────────┘
```

Sudden injuries can often be accompanied by shock. In such cases recovery and healing will happen most effectively in the hands of a capable person who can deal calmly with the situation. Prompt action and calmness are the most important factors in first aid. Having some knowledge of and practice in performing emergency resuscitation is also essential.

This guide serves as a very basic source of information that you can refer to in a crisis. It is strongly advised to complete a more advanced first aid training program through your local Red Cross or Heart Association. This guide is no substitute for a more complete and extensive first aid reference.

WHEN POSSIBLE, ALWAYS WASH YOUR HANDS THOROUGHLY WITH HOT SOAPY WATER BEFORE CARING FOR ANY OF THE CONDITIONS ON THE FOLLOWING PAGES.

BURNS

DESCRIPTION

Burns are tissue injuries caused by heat, chemicals, electricity, or irradiation.

a) First degree burns affect the superficial layers of the skin and cause reddening of affected tissue. The burned skin blanches with pressure.

b) Second degree burns affect varying layers of skin, which form red, tender blisters.

c) Third degree burns destroy the full thickness of the underlying tissue and skin. The burned skin is tough and leathery and is usually not tender.

ACTION

a) Immediately pour cold water over the affected parts and continue to do so for several minutes or until the pain begins to subside. This will help prevent blistering and keep the surrounding clothing from sticking to the skin. Do not apply ice.

b) Remove clothing only where necessary to see where the burn is.

c) Cover all burned areas with a clean dry cloth or sheet.

d) Remove all rings, watches, etc. from injured extremities to avoid a tourniquet effect.

f) If it is a severe burn, or if burns cover more than five percent of the body surface, take the person to the hospital.

g) Minor burns can be cared for at home with home remedies.[24]

HOME REMEDIES

See Section Eight for more information on the following:

Combudoron Gel

CUTS AND WOUNDS

DESCRIPTION

This section includes small cuts, skinned knees, and gaping wounds.

ACTION

a) Small cuts or puncture wounds should be allowed to bleed for a few seconds. Then apply a sterile gauze or bandage.

b) Skinned knees can be cleaned gently with fresh water and some sterile cotton or cotton balls. Allow the abrasion to dry in the air. A bandage may be necessary to prevent rubbing of clothing. The bandage can be changed two or three times a week.

c) In treating gaping wounds and more severe cuts, first stop the flow of blood by applying pressure with a clean cloth or a clean hand. Wounds from which blood is flowing or spurting should be bound firmly with as clean a cloth as possible, but do not apply it so tightly that it becomes a tourniquet. Seek medical attention immediately.[25]

HOME REMEDIES

See Section Eight for more information on the following:

Calendula Ointment

Calendula Essence

FALLS

If a child or adult falls, watch for the following symptoms:

a) The person is probably fine if he or she begins to cry right away; no flat cushion-like swellings can be felt on the skull in the next 30 minutes or so; and once the person gets over the fright, he or she seems happy again.

b) Seek medical attention for a concussion or more severe injury if the person loses consciousness and starts vomiting or if flat, cushion-like swelling appears on the skull. Also, check for abnormality in the size of the pupils. Is the pupil of one eye more dilated than the other? Do the pupils respond to bright light? Can the person move his or her extremities in a normal manner? Is there a loss of coordination or dizziness? Is there blood or clear fluid draining from the ear or nose? Is there a severe, unrelenting headache?

IN THE CASE OF SERIOUS INJURY:

a) First listen to see if the person is breathing, speaks or moves. If so, turn them gently on their side, wrap the body warmly to prevent shock and stay by the person's side to provide a calm gentle presence until emergency medical care arrives.

b) If the person has lost consciousness, but is still breathing, do not move them until trained help comes, unless there is danger from fire or traffic.

c) If the person is not breathing, give artificial respiration. If there is no pulse or heart beat, begin heart massage.

d) If there are badly injured parts of the body, especially the back, DO NOT move to another position. This can cause more trauma. Cover the person, if possible, and wait until emergency care arrives.[26]

HOME REMEDIES

See Section Eight for more information on the following:

Arnica 6X

Arnica Ointment or Essence

INSECT BITES

DESCRIPTION

Insects may bite, sting, inject poison, invade tissue, or transmit disease. They can cause a wide range of reactions.

a) Local reactions are caused by tissue inflammation and destruction from local poison. Symptoms of local reactions include redness at the site of the sting, heat, swelling, itching, and blisters.

b) Toxic reactions are due to a large dose of the poison and can cause nausea, vomiting, headache, fever, diarrhea, fainting, drowsiness, muscle spasms, and convulsions.

c) Systemic or allergic reactions usually occur from a previous sensitization and can produce itching eyes, facial flushing, hives, dry cough, throat constriction, difficult or noisy breathing, abdominal cramps, chills, respiratory failure, cardiovascular difficulties and on rare occasions, death.[27]

ACTION

If a bee or other insect has injected its stinger into a blood vessel, or if the child has a known allergy:

a) Remove the stinger at once by scraping it out with a credit card or other flat, thin object. Do not squeeze it.

b) Seek immediate medical attention.

c) If you have a bee sting kit, use it. (Bee sting kits usually contain epinephrine to manage severe allergic reactions.)

d) Clean the wound.

e) Apply cold packs to the bite or sting, alternating 10 minutes on, then 10 minutes off.

f) Elevate and rest the affected part.

g) In severe allergic reactions oxygen or artificial respiration may be needed.

HOME REMEDIES

See Section Eight for more information on the following:

Onion

Combudoron

SPRAINS AND STRAINS

DESCRIPTION

A sprain is an injury to a ligament. A strain is a partial or complete disruption of the muscle or tendon. Strains are usually associated with overuse injuries, whereas sprains usually result from trauma like falls, twisting, or accidents. Symptoms include swelling, pain, redness or bruising, tenderness, walking with a limp, and decreased range of motion. If the pain and swelling last for more than two days it is good to have the problem checked by a healthcare professional.

ACTION

    a) Use the "RICE" therapy: rest, ice, compression, elevation.

    b) An elastic ACE bandage may provide comfort.

    c) Prevent motion of the affected area.[28]

An ankle or foot x-ray may be necessary if the following symptoms are present:

    a) Inability to bear weight on the foot.

    b) Bone tenderness on the bones or inner or outer ankle, not the soft tissue.

HOME REMEDIES

See Section Eight for more information on the following:

Arnica 6X

Arnica Ointment

8

A Reference Guide to Home Therapies

TEMPLATE

∞ **DESCRIPTION OF PLANT OR SUBSTANCE**

∞ **HEALING PROPERTIES**

∞ **COMMON USES**

∞ **PREPARATIONS AND INSTRUCTIONS FOR USE**

GENERAL DOSAGE GUIDELINES FOR USE OF REMEDIES AND NATURAL MEDICINES:

Dosage: If a symptom is very severe, take one dose every 15 minutes; then slowly cut back to one dose three times a day before meals. Do not stop taking the remedy until two or three days after the fever and symptoms are gone. The remedies must be given regularly and consistently if they are to work.

Pellets: Homeopathic pellets should be administered by tapping the dosage directly into the lid and tapping the pellets under the tongue, being careful not to touch the lid to the mouth. If possible, do not touch the pellets with your hands. The general rule of thumb for calculating proper dosages for children is one pellet per year of age. Adults can take up to 10 pellets. (See Fig. 8-1.)

Infants under 6 months:	one pellet
6 months to 2 years:	2 pellets
3 years:	3 pellets
4 years:	4 pellets
5 years:	5 pellets
Over 6 to adult	5 - 10 pellets

Fig. 8-1. Recommended dosages of homeopathic pellets.

Liquid: Remedies in liquid form are taken orally by putting the drops in a teaspoon of water. The daily dosage is identical to pellets. (i.e., one drop per year of age for children under 6. Then 5 - 10 drops for adults). Some liquid remedies are prepared with alcohol. If you are sensitive to alcohol, then try another form.

Tablets: Remedies in tablet form are to be taken orally and allowed to dissolve under the tongue. The dosage should be verified on the individual bottle.

Children tend to chew tablets. For infants, crush the tablet into a powder and moisten with a few drops of water on a spoon.

Powder: The dosage for powders is the same for all ages: a pea-sized portion on the handle of a teaspoon.[29]

Note: If you already have some of the following substances or prefer using others, that's fine. Many of the basic principles will still apply and can inspire you to create your own healing kit.

ARNICA

(Arnica montana)

DESCRIPTION

Arnica montana is a hardy perennial that grows between one and two feet tall. Its yellow, scented flowers bloom in the summer. The plant grows high up in the mountains and prefers a moist, cool environment. Its hairy quality indicates the presence of silica. The pattern of its roots also reveals the contracting and cold element present in arnica.

HEALING PROPERTIES

Arnica is most effective in cases where the internal fluid processes have exceeded their limits (e.g., swelling). It is also valuable in cases where there is loss of form or structure of the tissues. When it is applied, the essence of the arnica plant transfers a cooling quality to the body. The silica brings the form-creating forces to help the body reform or rebuild injured tissue.[30]

COMMON USES

Arnica is most commonly used for *internal* wounds, such as internal bleeding, swelling, and bruising. It can also aid in recovery from physical and emotional trauma. Use arnica for sprains, headaches, bruises, post-surgery or post-dentistry care, fractures, sore muscles, and post-partum care.

One mother writes: "Everyone with young children needs to stock arnica ointment! If applied immediately after a bump or scrape, it can take the pain away and greatly reduce the expected swelling and bruising. It's the closest thing to magic I've seen."

PREPARATIONS AND INSTRUCTIONS FOR USE

- **Arnica Essence**, in liquid form, should be used <u>externally only</u>. If the skin is broken, see Calendula.

  Arnica Compresses: Dilute one teaspoon of arnica essence in 1/2 cup of water or sprinkle 20 drops on a damp, cold gauze pad or washcloth. Wring out so that no drips will run down. Apply to the injury and hold for several minutes. The arnica essence is especially helpful in applying compresses to more severe injuries in areas like the head, where it is difficult to apply ointment.

  Arnica Wipes: These are individually wrapped for travel and home convenience.

- **Arnica 6X** can be taken immediately after the trauma. Continue every 15 to 30 minutes until severity subsides. Continue with one dose three times a day until a day or two after healing is complete.

- **Arnica Ointment** can be applied very frequently to bring healing to swelling, bruises, sprains, and sore, aching muscles.

CALENDULA

(Marigold or Calendula officinalis)

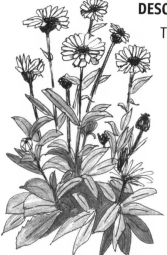

DESCRIPTION

The marigold originated in the Mediterranean countries, where it flowers throughout the year. Vivid orange flowers appear from the thick, round buds. The flowers open at sunrise and follow the movement of the sun to absorb its rays. In the evening the petals close up again. When they are to be used for medicinal purposes, the flowers should be picked early in the morning before they open. Marigolds are easily grown, but be certain that you have the calendula variety.

The unique and striking feature of this plant is the contrast between its rough, untidy leaves and its strictly developed flower. In this beautifully shaped flower, the plant conquers the chaotic, disorderly character typical of the leaves. It is this property of creating order that the marigold offers when used as a medicinal plant.

HEALING PROPERTIES

Calendula can stimulate wounds to heal, so new tissue can be formed. It is also an antiseptic with anti-inflammatory properties, so it promotes rapid healing.

COMMON USES

Calendula can help heal cuts and wounds, boils, inflamed wounds, hemorrhoids, and inflamed and painful varicose veins. See Cuts and Wounds in Section Seven.

PREPARATIONS AND INSTRUCTIONS FOR USE

FOR EXTERNAL USE ONLY!

- **Calendula Ointment** can be applied to a sterile gauze or bandage to cover a cleaned wound. Or simply apply the ointment directly to the cut with a sterile cotton swab. Remember to wash your hands thoroughly before and after application.

- **Calendula Essence** can be used as a compress to stimulate healing of more severe injuries.

  Calendula Compress:

  1) Always wash hands first with hot soapy water.

  2) Dilute calendula essence as described on package. (Usually about half a teaspoon in half a cup of fresh water is recommended.)

  3) Place a cotton cloth in the solution and wring slightly.

  4) Place a towel under the area to be treated and place the very damp cloth on the wound for 5 to 10 minutes or so. Some of the leftover calendula solution can be poured over the cloth to keep it from drying out.

  5) Throw away the used compress, and disinfect the bowl and other materials used for the treatment.

  6) After the wound has been cleaned in this way, watch for a small pink border to appear around the edge of the wound. This is an indication that new tissue is, in fact, being formed. Calendula ointment can be used between compress applications.[31]

CARBO BETULAE

(Plant charcoal from birch wood)

DESCRIPTION

The most distinguishing feature of the birch tree is its smooth, deadened, white bark. At the other end of the spectrum, it is one of the earliest trees to send forth its fresh, vital leaves in spring. It is the birch tree's mastery over these two polarities the death process and life process, that gives us insight into its healing capacities.

HEALING PROPERTIES

The essence of birch wood is its unique property of creating an open space as it pulls in two directions between the polarities of the bark and the leaves. The remedy, called carbo betulae, is prepared by charring the birch wood to create charcoal. We have all witnessed charcoal's ability to ignite, thereby showing its capacity to hold and absorb oxygen. This charred birch wood remedy possesses the extraordinary ability to absorb gases and toxins in the "space" created by the polarities and the oxygen-poor charring process.

COMMON USES

Carbo betulae can help relieve stomachache, indigestion, bloating, and diarrhea.

PREPARATIONS AND INSTRUCTIONS FOR USE

- **Carbo Betulae 3X:**

    DOSAGE: Take one tablet or pea-sized portion every one to two hours or until symptoms subside.

CHAMOMILE

(Matricaria chamomilla)

DESCRIPTION

The chamomile plant cannot survive in shade or a damp environment. Its feathery leaves allow the sun to shine right down to the root of the plant. The plant typically flowers profusely and for a long time from spring to fall. The round yellow head of the flower is hollow and contains a bubble of air. The volatile, etheric oil from the flowers has a blue color, not yellow or reddish yellow like most etheric oils.

The chamomile plant is so completely saturated with light, air, and sun. It is as if the chamomile plant "cramps up" to put such enormous energy into its sunny flowers.

HEALING PROPERTIES

This plant carries light, warmth, and air to heal and bring form to places in the body where there is a lot of secretion and breakdown of tissue. It also has an anti-cramping or antispasmodic effect that helps regulate or recreate balance.

COMMON USES

Chamomile can aid anxiety, nervous tension, stomachache, stubborn colds, bronchitis, bladder infections, toothache.

PREPARATIONS AND INSTRUCTIONS FOR USE

- **Brewing Chamomile:** (loose herb form)
    1) Boil a quart of fresh, cold water.
    2) Add a small handful of chamomile flowers.

3) Remove the pan from the heat, and let the herbs brew for about two minutes.

4) Pour the tea through a sieve into a cup or bowl.

Tea: For general anxiety and nervousness, drink one or two cups. Then lie down and rest for a short time.

A rinse with chamomile tea can also have a soothing effect on a toothache.

• **Abdominal Compresses:** These are used for bladder and kidney infections, stomachaches, menstrual cramps, and general digestive complaints.

1) Allow the ill person to go to the bathroom and then lie down on a bed. Make sure the person's feet are warm. Offer a warm-water bottle.

2) Make sure the room is comfortable.

3) Fold a piece of cotton or a cotton towel in half to just fit over the abdomen.

4) Immerse the cotton a bowl of hot brewed chamomile.

5) Wring it out completely so that it will not drip.

6) Quickly apply the cotton compress, as hot as the person can stand it.

7) Quickly cover the compress with another piece of cotton cloth or woolen fabric.

8) Apply a hot-water bottle (with just a little water) over the stomach or bladder to keep it warm.

9) Cover the person thoroughly so that his or her shoulders and feet are tucked in.

10) The cloths will stay warm and can be left in place for 20 to 30 minutes.

11) If the person falls asleep, let the cloths stay on and dry out by themselves.

12) If the cloths are removed, the person should stay tucked in and should rest for at least half an hour.

- **Inhalations:** These steam treatments can bring relief to colds, coughs, and sinus and bronchial congestion

  When inhaled, the vapor of the chamomile has a warming and healing effect on the mucous membranes of the nose and throat.

  1) Place a handful of chamomile flowers in a bowl.

  2) Pour a quart of boiling water on the flowers.

  3) Place the bowl on a table or in a sink.

  4) Have the person lean over the bowl. Cover the bowl and the person's head with a large towel or sheet. Make sure that no air can enter from the outside. (When leaning over the bowl, the person inhaling the vapor should be careful not to lean too close to the steam, as it can burn the face.)

  5) The inhalation treatment can last 10 to 20 minutes.

  6) Remove the bowl and sheet, and place a dry towel around the person's head and forehead to prevent cooling down too quickly.

  7) Have the person lie down for 30 minutes after being tucked in warmly.

- **Compresses:** To soothe toothaches or other painful spots try the following.

  1) Place a teaspoon of chamomile flowers in a small piece of gauze or thin cloth and fold. (A ready-to-use chamomile tea bag can also be used if you are in a hurry and have one on hand.)

  2) Place the compress in a sieve, and hold it over the steam of boiling water to moisten the flowers.

  3) Place the compress over the painful area or between the gum and the cheek.[32]

CINNABAR

(Mercuric sulfide, a naturally occurring mineral)

DESCRIPTION

Mercury is an interesting metal in that it is liquid-like yet silvery, heavy, and nearly solid. The character or essence of this metal is to act as a mediator--not quite liquid, not quite solid. It helps in moving an illness process from one state to another. It must be "potentized" or greatly diluted to render it non-toxic and to free its healing properties.

It is well known that sulfur is very loosely bound to living substances, as noted in how readily it is freed when a living organism dies; the foul smell of decomposition is the release of sulfur. It is readily combustible, ready to give forth to the air and release its inner warmth. It reminds us of the metabolic pole and the source of the warmth production. Sulfur is also known for its ability to detoxify poisons, much like the metabolic/digestive system's detoxifier, the liver.

HEALING PROPERTIES

Mercury, the mediator, combined with the warmth of sulfur creates cinnabar, a red substance that helps move a red-hot inflammatory process back into a healthy balance.

COMMON USES

Cinnabar is most helpful in cases of the common cold accompanied by sore throat. DO NOT use it if there is pus in the back of the throat.

PREPARATIONS AND INSTRUCTIONS FOR USE

- **Cinnabar Powder** is made from a "potentized" combination of cinnabar, belladonna, and apis venenum perum.

DOSAGE: Take one pea-sized portion every two hours at the onset of symptoms. Gradually reduce to the same dosage three times a day for duration of illness, continuing one or two days after its resolution.

COMBUDORON GEL

(Stinging nettle or Urtica urens and Arnica montana)

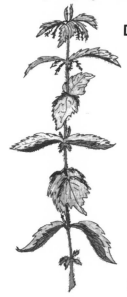

DESCRIPTION

The leading ingredient in combudoron is made from the small stinging nettle plant which does not grow higher than 20 inches. The most striking thing about the plant is its leaves. The leaves of the small stinging nettle have a fairly rounded shape with a short tip with serrated edges. The stinging hairs on the leaves release a fierce, corrosive fluid when they are touched, causing a burning, itchy rash on the skin.

HEALING PROPERTIES

The flower of the small stinging nettle plant is generally an expression of heat, which can only be felt when the plant is touched. Thus, its medicinal quality lies in its ability to encompass heat when administered.

The homeopathic principle of "like cures like" is employed in the medicinal use of the stinging nettle.

COMMON USES

Combudoron can be used for burns, insect bites, itchy skin rashes (hives and shingles), and sunburn. See Burns and Insect Bites in Section Five.

PREPARATIONS AND INSTRUCTIONS FOR USE

In case of burns, always remember to immediately place the affected area under cold water for a least five minutes. Watch to be sure that the patient does not faint.

- **Combudoron Gel** should be applied to the affected area fairly thickly so that the protective gauze applied over it does not stick. If this does happen, do not tear the gauze off. Simply apply more gel over the piece of gauze, and it will automatically separate from the skin at a later point. In more minor cases, a thin layer of gel may be applied, creating a protective film as it dries.

COTTAGE CHEESE

(Curd cheese)

DESCRIPTION

Curd cheese is made by leaving fresh milk to separate and sour. As curd cheese dries out, it produces a "suction effect," creating a space where an equilibrium can develop.

HEALING PROPERTIES

Cottage cheese brings balance to inflamed processes (bronchitis, boils, mastitis). In the case of mastitis, the compress soothes the pain and the sour substance dissipates the infection as it dries up.

COMMON USES

Cottage cheese can aid in the healing of bronchitis, mastitis, swollen joints, and boils.

PREPARATIONS AND INSTRUCTIONS FOR USE

Breast Compress for Mastitis

(Important: See notes under Mastitis before using this compress.)

1) Wash your hands.

2) Iron a piece of cotton to eliminate the danger of infection.

3) Place the clean cotton cloth on a towel, and apply cold cottage cheese or quark with a sterile spoon. The amount of curd depends on the size of the breast and the inflammation. The compress should amply cover the area.

4) Fold the edges of the cloth and apply to the breast so that only one layer of cloth is between the curd and the skin.

5) The curd cheese will dry out after 20 minutes. Immediately remove the compress, and rinse the cloth in cold water. The compress must be removed after a maximum of 20 minutes to prevent it from becoming warm and actually stimulating the inflammation.

6) This process can be repeated once or twice a day. In more severe cases, repeat after each feeding.

Compress for Boils

1) Wash your hands thoroughly before and after the application.

2) Warm the curd and spread it in a small compress made of clean cotton cloth.

3) Apply the compress to the affected area.

4) The compress may be covered with a warm-water bottle for no more than 20 minutes at a time.[33]

ECHINACEA

(Echinacea angustifolia or purple coneflower)

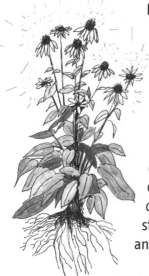

DESCRIPTION

Echinacea is one of the coneflowers, a group of native American wildflowers from the daisy family. It is characterized by spiny flowering heads with an elevated receptacle which forms a cone. The tall stalks reach to the sun and are covered with coarse hairs. The bluish red color of the cone-like flower mirrors the bluish red color of a boil which has progressed to a stage where it is about to point, but stops and does not suppurate (burst).

HEALING PROPERTIES

Echinacea stimulates the production of white cells that help promote healing. It enhances the body's ability to eliminate unwanted bacteria and damaged cells. Echinacea also helps protect cells during infection, and it prevents pathogens, bacteria, and viruses from entering in the first place.[34]

COMMON USES

Echinacea aids in healing inflammation and fever associated with colds, flu, sore throat, bladder and kidney infections, infected wounds, burns, pneumonia and bronchitis.

PREPARATIONS AND INSTRUCTIONS FOR USE

- **Echinacea Compound** is an effective combination of substances that are all useful in the healing of viral illnesses (especially cold and flu symptoms) and in cases of compromised immunity. The compound includes Lachesis mutus, Echinacea angustifola, Equisetum arvense, Vespa crabro, Apis mellifica, Baptisia tinctoria, Thuja occidentalis.

DOSAGE:

Adults: Take five drops every hour at onset of symptoms or in very early stages of illness.

Children: See dosage chart at beginning of Section Eight.

Reduce dosage to three times a day (before meals) during illness and continue one or two days after the symptoms have resolved.

EUCALYPTUS

(Eucalyptus globulus)

DESCRIPTION

The eucalyptus tree is native to Australia and has been transplanted to marshy districts in mild climates because of its ability to absorb water. The volatile oil possesses a remarkable ability to convert water, in the presence of air and sunlight, into hydrogen peroxide.

HEALING PROPERTIES

The volatile oils of the eucalyptus plant have extraordinary deodorizing and antiseptic healing properties.

COMMON USES

Eucalyptus is most commonly used as an inhalation for chest colds, flu, bronchitis and asthma, mucous congestion, and sinusitis. It can also be used as a massage oil for a chest rub and in treating certain rheumatic conditions.

PREPARATIONS AND INSTRUCTIONS FOR USE

- **Eucalyptus Oil** is prepared from the essential volatile oil of the eucalyptus plant.

    Inhalation:

    1) Place a few drops of eucalyptus oil in a bowl.
    2) Add a quart of boiling water.
    3) Place the bowl on a table or in a sink.
    4) Have the person to be treated lean over the bowl. Cover the bowl and the person's head with a large towel or sheet. Make sure that no air can enter from the outside. When leaning over the bowl, be careful

that the person's face does not to come too close to the steam, as it can burn.

5) The inhalation treatment can last 5 to 20 minutes.

6) Remove the bowl and sheet, and place a dry towel around the person's head and forehead to prevent cooling down too quickly.

7) Have the person lie down for 30 minutes after being tucked in warmly.

Vaporizer: A few drops can be added to the vaporizer to clean the air and bring healing qualities to the lungs and nasal passages.

Rub or massage: Add a few drops to a good olive or almond oil, and rub into chest and back. Cover with a warm cloth as desired. Be careful to try a small test patch first to see if the skin is sensitive.

INFLUDORON

(Ferrum phosphoricum or phosphate of iron)

DESCRIPTION

The significant quality of this remedy is the powerful synergy of the combined remedies, which are all directed toward treating the symptomology of the flu.

HEALING PROPERTIES

As discussed earlier, our blood is enriched by iron (ferrum) which is the carrier of oxygen and mediator of human consciousness. Phosphorus is a mineral uniquely capable of combining with water to give off its inner light. In the remedy form, ferrum phosphoricum directs "inner light" and consciousness to inflamed areas in the head area, the seat of greatest consciousness. This carrier of "inner light" circumvents the need for fever. It also strengthens the host's immune response by increasing the oxygen supply to head-centered inflammations such as colds or flus.

COMMON USES

Infludoron can bring relief to flus and head or chest colds.

PREPARATIONS AND INSTRUCTIONS FOR USE

- **Infludoron** is a homeopathically prepared pellet form of ferrum phosphoricum, Aconitum naapellus, bryonia, Eucalyptus globulus, Eupatorium perfoliatum, and sabadilla.

  ### DOSAGE:

  Adults: One dose (5 to 10 pellets) every two hours at onset. Reduce to one dosage three times a day before meals, and continue for one or two days after the symptoms resolve.

  Children: See dosage chart at the beginning of Section Eight.

LAVENDER

(Lavandula angustifolia)

DESCRIPTION

In summer, the lavender plant changes dramatically as it moves into the flowering stage. Its beautiful blue flowers are so predominant that they almost penetrate back down into the stem. This is shown by the bluish color of the stem.

During its flowering stage, lavender produces one of the noblest scents in the plant world. It is clean and soothing by nature.

HEALING PROPERTIES

Lavender helps free the emotions from overactivity. It also strengthens and calms the nerves, relaxes spasms, counteracts faintness, and can bring sleep.[35]

COMMON USES

Lavender can bring relief to stress-related headaches, restlessness with high fever, sciatica, and general nervousness. It can also bring rapid pain relief when it is applied directly on minor burns.

PREPARATIONS AND INSTRUCTIONS FOR USE

- **Lavender Oil** is the volatile oil extracted from the lavender plant.

  Baths and Soaks: Put 5 to 10 drops of the oil in a bath. One or two drops may be added to a warm bowl of water to wash hands or gently wipe the face and body. The oil can also be added to a bowl of healing water to soak a bump or wound. Lavender bathmilks are also available.

Antiseptic: Using a Q-tip, dab lavender oil directly onto bites, stings, burns, sores and scar tissue.

LEMON
(Citrus media)

DESCRIPTION

When we examine the lemon plant in its totality, we can notice that the outward-turned character of the flowers is reversed in the fruit. The plant is metamorphosed into a strictly ordered, contracting process. When used for medicinal purposes, the lemon repeats this process in conditions where excessive heat processes need to be limited and restrained.

HEALING PROPERTIES

Compresses with lemon juice can be applied on the feet and lower parts of the legs of a person with a high fever. The lemon helps guide the excessive heat in the head back down to the legs and helps disperse the heat as well. In cases of cold and sore throat, this treatment also leads the excessive metabolic activity from the nose and throat back to the lower regions.

COMMON USES

Lemon can be helpful in cases of high fever, bronchitis, sore throat, cough, and colds.

PREPARATIONS AND INSTRUCTIONS FOR USE

Cool Lemon Leg Compresses (for high fever):

Important Note! This compress should only be applied if the lower legs and feet are warm or hot to the touch.

1) Fill a bowl with lukewarm water.

2) Cut a lemon in half under the water and squeeze the juice out. This way both the juice and the etheric oil from the peel are released into the water.

3) Roll up two long, thin strips of cotton cloth and place them the bowl.

4) Have the person lie back comfortably and place a towel under each leg.

5) Thoroughly wring out the compresses, and wind one cotton strip around each leg from toe to knee.

6) Wrap each leg with a towel.

7) After 20 minutes the compresses will have dried out. (If not, they might have been too wet when wrung out.)

8) If the person falls into a peaceful sleep, the compresses can be left on, provided they have dried out.

9) This process can be repeated immediately or as often as needed to bring a high fever down to a more comfortable level.

Warm Lemon Throat Compress (for sore throat) or Chest Compress (for bronchitis, cough, and chest cold):

1) Pour boiling water into a bowl, and cut a lemon in half with a knife and fork.

2) Press out the two halves of the lemon using the base of a cup, to release the juice and etheric oils.

3) Place a folded strip of cotton cloth in the bowl and leave it to soak for a few minutes.

4) Wring the cotton strip out quickly and thoroughly by rolling it inside another cloth or hand towel and wringing it again.

5) Before applying the compress, always test it by touching the cotton to the person's skin to see if it is

too hot. Then roll the cotton around the person's neck or chest.

6) Place another cloth (if possible, a woolen one; otherwise cotton will do) over the compress, and fasten with a safety pin.

7) Have the person put on a warm pajama top and rest, tucked in to bed for 20 to 30 minutes.

8) If the cloth has become cold or the person feels uncomfortable before the twenty to thirty minutes have passed, then remove the cloth right away.

9) Have the person rest a bit after the compress has been removed.

Cool Lemon Foot Compress (for colds): This simple method is very effective in relieving irritation of the mucous membranes of the nose and throat.

1) Place thin slices of lemon on the soles of the feet.

2) Keep the slices in place with a bandage or strip of cotton.

3) Cover the feet and compresses with a woolen sock.

4) The compresses can be left in place all night and repeated nightly as necessary.[36]

Lemon, Milk, and Egg Nutrient Bath (for depletion): If a prolonged illness results in extended loss of appetite, weight loss, or general need for revitalization, the following bath can help replace nutrients and strengthen the life forces.

Ingredients include one lemon, one cup of milk, one egg.

1) Prepare the bathroom, attending to warmth and lighting. Also, remember to have warm pajamas or a blanket and maybe a hot-water bottle ready as soon as the bath is complete. A candle can be nice too.

2) Prepare a warm, comfortable bath (approximately 37 C. or 98.6 F. is the temperature at which human life

processes take place). If the bath is too hot, it can be depleting.

3) Cut the lemon in half under the water, and squeeze out the juice.

4) Whisk the milk and egg together in a cup before adding them to the bath water.

5) Blend the ingredients into the bath water by moving your hand in a slow, rhythmic, figure-eight motion. If it suits you, focus on a couple of positive thoughts about what a healed state would look like, while you are at it. Why not?

6) Have the person stay in the bath for 20 to 30 minutes.

7) Tuck the person into a warm bed to rest for a time afterwards.

LEVISTICUM

(Lovage)

DESCRIPTION

Levisticum has a short main root with several long roots branching down. These long, tough, resistant roots enable it to deeply "inhale" from the earth. It has a limited ability to "exhale", as shown by its small flowers. So it spends most of the year confined to the form of its strongest part: the root. The root has an exceptionally volatile, aromatic oil and a liquid resin.

HEALING PROPERTIES

Levisticum's extraordinary ability to inhale deeply into its root can help drive out watery inflammation. In the case of ear infection, for example, the watery substance is replaced with the ear's natural environment, air. Levisticum can also help regenerate new tissue.

COMMON USES

Levisticum is commonly used to aid in the healing of ear infections.

PREPARATIONS AND INSTRUCTIONS FOR USE

- **Levisticum** is prepared from the lovage root in a "potentized" pellet form. It is usually used in a homeopathically prepared potency of 3X. Levisticum is available by prescription only.

  DOSAGE: Take the appropriate dose every 15 minutes in cases accompanied by severe pain, and decrease the frequency as pain subsides. Since ear infections take a long time to heal, it is helpful to continue taking the remedy for several days or even weeks after the acute symptoms have subsided.

ONION

(Allium cepa)

DESCRIPTION

The strength of the onion is revealed in the layers of the bulb with its high content of sulfur, and especially in its powerfully formed root.

HEALING PROPERTIES

Onion has the ability to control the abundance of sulfur and stimulate the metabolic processes. These activities can help to overcome inflammations in the head and chest area in humans, which corresponds to the area where the bulb of the onion grows between the roots and leaves.

COMMON USES

Onion can be used to aid in the healing of earaches, insect bites, and inflammations.

PREPARATIONS AND INSTRUCTIONS FOR USE

In general, an onion compress will quickly reduce pain. If this does not occur, you may need to consult your healthcare provider.

- **Onion Compress**

  For Earache:

  1) Dice a fresh yellow or white onion into very small pieces.

  2) Place the onion pieces in the middle of a piece of cloth or gauze and fold several times so that no onion falls out. (Alternate method: It is also possible to

squeeze the juice out of the onion with a garlic press onto a piece of cotton.)

3) Place the compress on or behind the ear, and hold it in place with a bandage.

4) For small children, it may be easier to just hold the compress on their ear and cover it with a cap that covers the ears. It may also be held on with cling gauze.

5) Leave the compress on for a few hours or until it no longer smells.

6) NOTE: Skin irritation may occur if the compress is pressed down too firmly on the skin.

For Joints:

For an inflammation of a joint or ligament, it is possible to use a large onion.

1) Remove the outer layers of the onion.

2) Bruise the onion layers slightly, and place them on the skin so that they overlap one another.

3) Use a bandage to keep the layers in place.[37]

For Insect Bites:

To care for minor insect bites, remove the stinger at once, and apply a freshly cut slice of onion or cool, wet onion compress onto the affected area.

AFTERWORD

Getting sick can be very scary. It can bring out our worst sides and stir up the parts of our lives that need attention. Sometimes we just want to turn and run.

We hope that this book can be of comfort during those times. May it serve as a source of practical advice and information to help you accomplish the hands-on part of getting well and staying well. In time, we hope your positive experiences with healing will teach you how these scary moments can be turned into rich opportunities to reconnect with your self, with your loved ones, and your sense of purpose.

As you use this book, please let us know where it may be improved. Tell us your experiences. What parts of the book have you found helpful? We look forward to hearing from you. Send your replies by mail to:

Healing at Home Resources, P.O. Box 2622, Ann Arbor, MI 48106 or e-mail: lindo@compuserve.com

Best wishes.

RESOURCES

HOME REMEDIES

    Dr. Possum's World, 4455 Torrance Blvd., #270, Torrance, CA 90503; (800) 827-4086. A mail order catalog with a variety of holistic healing products and books for the whole family.

    Homecare Essentials, 12525 Parish Rd., San Diego, CA 92128; (619) 673-5975. Beautiful, handmade natural fiber supplies for homecare treatments and external applications.

    Cascade HealthCare Products, Inc., 141 Commercial Street, N.E., Salem, OR 97301; (800) 443-9942; website: www.1cascade.com   Cascade offers a wide variety of healing substances including supplies for the healing kit. They also have an extensive book and video catalog.

The following are three very high caliber companies that offer a variety of healing products.

    WALA - Raphael Pharmacy, 7957 California Avenue, Fair Oaks, CA 95628; (800) 677-0015.

    Weleda Pharmacy, 175 North Route 9W, Congers, NY 10920; (800) 241-1030; e-mail: info@weleda.com; Internet: www.usa.weleda.com

    Uriel Pharmacy, N8464 Sterman Rd., East Troy, WI 53120; (414) 642-2858; e-mail: uriel@elknet.net

HEALING AND ILLNESS

    American Association for Naturopathic Physicians, 2366 Eastlake Ave., Suite 322, Seattle, WA 98102.

    American Holistic Medical Association and American Holistic Nurses Association, 4101 Lake Bone Trail, Suite 201, Raleigh, NC 27607.

    Anthroposophical Nurses Association of America, 215 E. Main St., Elkton, NC 21921.

Informed Home Birth, P.O. Box 1733, Fair Oaks, CA 95628.

National Vaccine Information Center, 512 W. Maple Ave., Suite 206, Vienna, VA 22180.

Physicians Association for Anthroposophical Medicine (PAAM), 1923 Geddes Rd., Ann Arbor, MI 48104; (734) 662-9355.

Process Acupressure Unlimited, P.O. Box 1096, Capitola, CA 95010; (831) 475-3124.

The Process Work Center, 2049 N.W. Hoyt, Portland, OR 97209; (503) 223-8188.

PUBLISHERS

Anthroposophic Press, 3390 Route 9, Hudson, NY 12534; (518) 851-2054.

Mercury Press, 241 Hungry Hollow Rd., Chestnut Ridge, NY, 10977; (914) 425-9357.

NOTES

Section One

1. John Thompson, *Natural Childhood* (New York: Simon & Schuster Inc., 1994), pp. 44-46.

2. Sally Fallon, *Nourishing Traditions : The Cookbook that Challenges Politically Correct Nutrition and Diet Dictocrats* (San Diego: Promotion Publishing, 1995).

Section Two

3. Aminah Raheem, *Soul Return* (Lower Lake, CA: Aslan Publishing, 1987).

4. Philip Incao, M.D., *Patient Handout.*

5. Karen Sullivan, *Natural Home Remedies* (Rockport, MA: Element Books, 1997), p. 24.

6. Philip Incao, M.D., *op.cit.*

7. Michaela Gloekler and Wolfgang Goebel, *A Guide to Child Health* (Hudson, NY: Anthroposophic Press, Inc., 1990), p. 32.

Section Three

8. Philip Incao, M.D., *op.cit.*

9. Thomas Cowan, M.D., *Patient Handout.*

10. Thomas Cowan, M.D., *op.cit.*

11. Philip Incao, M.D., *op.cit.*

12. Clinton Greenstone, M.D., *Patient Handout.*

13. T. Bentheim, *Caring for the Sick at Home* (Hudson, NY: Anthroposophic Press, Inc., 1987), pp. 34-36.

14. Otto Wolf, *Home Remedies* (Hudson, NY: Anthroposophic Press, Inc., 1984), p.11.

15. Mary Carmichael, *Lilipoh,* Vol. 14, Issue 12, 1998, p. 26.

16. W.J. McIsaac, "Reconsidering Sore Throat, Part 2: Alternative Approach and Practical Office Tools," *Canadian Family Physician,* 43:495-500, March 1997.

Section Four

17. D.N. McKay, "Treatment of Acute Bronchitis in Adults Without Underlying Lung Disease," *Journal of General Internal Medicine,* 11C95: 557-62, Sept. 1996.

18. J.O. Hendley, "Editorial comment: The host response, not the virus, causes the symptoms of the common cold." *Clin Infect Dis*, April 1998, 26:847-8.

19. P. Little, "Reattendance and Complications in a Randomized Trial of Prescribing Strategies for Sore Throat," *BMJ.* 315(7104): 350-2, Aug. 9, 1997.

20. Philip Incao, M.D., *op.cit.*

21. Michaela Gloekler and Wolfgang Goebel, *op.cit.,* pp. 39-40.

22. C. Del Mar et al., "Are antibiotics indicated as initial treatment for children with acute otitis media? A meta-analysis," *BMJ* 314:1526-9, 1997.

23. Michaela Gloekler and Wolfgang Goebel, *op.cit.*, p. 26.

Section Five

24. Michaela Gloekler and Wolfgang Goebel, *op.cit.*, p. 397.

25. Michaela Gloekler and Wolfgang Goebel, *op.cit.*, p. 399.

26. Michaela Gloekler and Wolfgang Goebel, *op.cit.*, p. 397.

27. Mark Dambro, M.D., *The Five Minute Health Advisor* (Baltimore, MD: Williams and Wilkins, Inc., 1997), pp. 262-265.

28. Mark Dambro, M.D., *op.cit.*, p. 446.

Section Six

29. Philip Incao, M.D., *op.cit.*

30. T. Bentheim, *op.cit.*, p. 65.

31. T. Bentheim, *op.cit.*, p. 83.

32. T. Bentheim, *op.cit.*, pp. 87-95.

33. T. Bentheim, *op.cit.*, pp. 87-95.

34. Christopher Hobbs, "Echinacea - The Immune Herb" (Santa Cruz, CA: Botanica Press, 1996), p. 12.

35. Wilhelm Pelikan, *Healing Plants* (Spring Valley, NY: Mercury Press, 1988), p. 42.

36. T. Bentheim, *op.cit.*, pp. 75-80.

37. T. Bentheim, *op.cit.*, pp. 111-114.

FURTHER READING

FAMILY RHYTHMS

Lifeways: Working with Family Questions by Gudrun Davey and Bons Voors is a helpful collection of essays by various authors on children, family life, and balancing parenting with personal fulfillment. Although one major section of the book is devoted specifically to Christian festivals, the remainder of the book should be an inspiration to all. (Stroud, UK: Hawthorn Press, 1983)

Seven Times the Sun by Shea Darian is an excellent source of gentle inspiration for developing family rhythms through song, story, rhythm and ritual. (San Diego: Lura Media, 1984)

HEALING AND ILLNESS

A Guide to Child Health by M. Glockler and W. Goebel offers a deeper resource for caring for the health of the whole child: mind, body, and spirit. It is a unique look at childhood illnesses, healthy development, and education. (Hudson, NY: Anthroposophic Press, 1984)

A Slice of Life by Lee Sturgeon Day is a compelling and very personal story of healing through breast cancer. (Royal Oak, MI: Lifeways, 1991)

Anthroposophical Medicine Today by R. Leviton is a very clear and simple discussion of the fruits of anthroposophical medicine. Woven throughout is a woman's personal story of healing and transformation and her battle with lupus. Highly recommended! (Hudson, NY: Anthroposophic Press, 1984)

Caring for the Sick at Home by T. Bentheim brings a deeper look at home care and treatment of the sick for lay people and professionals. It is also a very practical guide to working with external applications. (Hudson, NY: Anthroposophic Press, 1984)

Choices In Healing by Michael Lerner is an invaluable guide to integrating the best of conventional and complementary approaches to cancer. (Cambridge: MIT Press, 1994)

Fever, Its History, Cause and Function by E. Atkins offers a deeper insight into the value of fever. (The Yale Journal of Biology and Medicine, 55, 1982)

How to Raise a Healthy Child in Spite of Your Doctor by R. Mendelsohn, M.D. is an easy-to-read, well-indexed reference to safe guidelines in caring for common childhood illnesses. (Chicago: Contemporary Books, 1984)

LILIPOH, Life Liberty and the Pursuit of Happiness Through Health is a journal that provides a forum for many different kinds of healing therapies. It is very family friendly and offers a wealth of practical information. (P.O. Box 649, Nyack, NY 10960 or lilipoh@aol.com)

LET YOUR HOME FEED YOUR SOUL

Shelter for the Spirit by Victoria Moran is a beautifully written invitation to bring simplicity and mindfulness to the home, the place that revives and nurtures us. It also offers practical advice and information on working, educating your children, and giving birth at home. (New York: Harper Collins, 1997)

The Non Toxic Home by Debra Lynn Dadd offers a wealth of information on a variety of household products from cleansers to bed linens to help protect yourself and your family from everyday toxins and health hazards. (Los Angeles: Jeremy Tarcher, Inc., 1986)

NUTRITION

Nourishing Traditions by Sally Fallon is far more than an excellent cookbook. It recalls the culinary wisdom and customs of our ancestors to guide us toward wise food choices and proper food preparation. (San Diego: Promotion Publishing, 1995)

Serving Fire by Anne Scott is an offering of rhythms and rituals of the hearth. It touches our need for nourishment that lies deep in our souls. (Berkeley, CA: Celestial Arts, 1994)

The Womanly Art of Breastfeeding by La Leche League International is an excellent source of support and information for the breastfeeding family. (New York: Penguin Books, 1991)

Whole Foods for the Whole Family by Roberta Johnson is a cookbook from La Leche League International. Contains over 900 recipes, using only whole unprocessed foods and minimal amounts of salt and sweeteners. The book also contains a Kids' Cookbook section. (Franklin Park, IL: La Leche League International, 1981)

PARENTING AND CHILD DEVELOPMENT

Endangered Minds: Why Children Don't Think and What We Can Do About It by Jane Healy is about how our present day life-style prevents children from learning and developing their full potential. (New York: Simon and Schuster, 1991)

Evolution's End by Joseph Chilton Pearce outlines five common practices in our society that hinder us from reaching our evolving potential: synthetic growth hormones, premature formal education, television, daycare, and hospital birth. (New York: Harper Collins, 1992)

Natural Childhood by John Thomson is one of the best really practical and holistic guides for parents of the developing child. (New York: Simon and Schuster, Inc., 1994)

You Are Your Child's First Teacher by Rahima Baldwin Dancy is a "must read" for every new parent. It can help set the tone for the first seven years giving parents insight into parenting and child development as inspired by Rudolf Steiner. (Berkeley, CA: Celestial Arts, 1989)

PERSONAL AND SPIRITUAL TRANSFORMATION

Blessed by Illness by L.F.C. Mees, M.D. envisions that the human beings and human evolution are large enough to include "illness" as an essential part of being human. By working *with* symptoms and ailments, not against them, we can come to true healing. (Hudson, NY: Anthroposophic Press, 1990)

Eastern Body Western Mind by Anodea Judith introduces psychology and the chakra system as a path to self. It realizes the spiritual nature of personality development within the logic of the body. (Berkeley, CA: Celestial Arts, 1996)

Soul Return by Aminah Raheem. is an exceptional book that explains the role spirituality plays in psychology. It also takes a practical look at how working with bodily symptoms and energy systems combined with love, wisdom, service, and enlightenment can lead to optimal health. (Lower Lake, CA: Aslan Publishing, 1987)

The Shaman's Body by Arnold Mindell has been described as "A new shamanism for transforming health, relationships and community." (New York: Simon and Schuster, 1991)

Working on Yourself Alone by Arnold Mindell offers a practical guide to unraveling the messages behind symptoms through process-oriented meditation, and dreamwork. It offers a pathway to those wanting a deeper understanding of themselves and their place in the world. (New York: Simon and Schuster, 1990)

SHARING NATURE

Earthways by Carole Petrash is filled with hands-on nature crafts and seasonal activities to enhance environmental awareness. (Rainier, MD: Gryphon House, Inc., 1992)

Sharing Nature With Children and *Sharing the Joy of Nature* by Jospeh Cornell include activities of nature awareness for parent and child, with an age-appropriate guide. (Nevada City, CA: Dawn Publications, 1979/ 1989)

SINGING

American Folk Songs for Children by Ruth Crawford Seager is an illustrated collection of over 90 folksongs for the whole family to enjoy, including work songs, ballads, chants and spirituals. (New York: Doubleday & Co., Inc., 1948)

Rise Up Singing edited by Peter Blood Patterson is an inspirational offering of lyrics to over 1200 songs, old and new, for lively musical gatherings. (Bethlehem, PA: Sing Out Corporation, 1988)

Pentatonic Songs by Elizabeth Lebret is a collection of songs especially appropriate for children from nursery through second grade .(Thornhill, Ontario: The Waldorf School Association of Ontario, 1985)

Shake It to the One That You Love the Best: Play Songs and Lullabies from Black Musical Traditions collected and adapted by Charyl Warren Mattox is a wonderful collection of timeless favorites. (El Sobrante, CA: Warren Mattox Production, 1989)

VACCINATIONS

How to Raise a Healthy Child in Spite of Your Doctor by R. Mendelsohn, M.D. is an easy to read, well-indexed reference to safe guidelines in caring for common childhood illnesses. It has an excellent section on the vaccination question. (Chicago: Contemporary Books, 1984)

Should I Have My Child Vaccinated? (Anthroposophical Medicine Association in the U.K., Rudolf Steiner House, 35 Park Road, London, NW1 6XT)

The Case Against Immunizations by R. Moskowitz, (The National Center for Homeopathy, 1500 Massachusetts Avenue NW, Washington, D.C., 20005)

Vaccinations: Concerns and Alternatives Sourcepack by Patty Brennan. (128 N. 7th St., Ann Arbor, MI 48103 or gbrennan@umich.edu)

Index